Nathan Dean, a native of Elizabethton, Tennessee, received a B.S. from the University of North Carolina at Chapel Hill and a Ph.D. from Cambridge University. As a physics professor at Iowa State University, he developed methods to model the behavior of quarks; after moving into university administration, he kept on modelling everything in sight, from competitive swimming to the coronavirus pandemic. Now retired from academe, he lives with his wife, Mary, in Atlanta.

This book is dedicated to all those who, like me, have spent their lives wishing they weighed less.

Nathan Dean

EXPONENTIAL WEIGHT LOSS

Easier than Dieting, and It Works!

AUSTIN MACAULEY PUBLISHERS™
LONDON • CAMBRIDGE • NEW YORK • SHARJAH

Copyright © Nathan Dean 2023

All rights reserved. No part of this publication may be reproduced, distributed, or transmitted in any form or by any means, including photocopying, recording, or other electronic or mechanical methods, without the prior written permission of the publisher, except in the case of brief quotations embodied in critical reviews and certain other non-commercial uses permitted by copyright law. For permission requests, write to the publisher.

Any person who commits any unauthorized act in relation to this publication may be liable to criminal prosecution and civil claims for damages.

The story, the experiences, the figures, and the words are the author's alone.

Ordering Information
Quantity sales: Special discounts are available on quantity purchases by corporations, associations, and others. For details, contact the publisher at the address below.

Publisher's Cataloging-in-Publication data
Dean, Nathan
Exponential Weight Loss

ISBN 9781649796622 (Paperback)
ISBN 9781649796639 (ePub e-book)

Library of Congress Control Number: 2023906370

www.austinmacauley.com/us

First Published 2023
Austin Macauley Publishers LLC
40 Wall Street 33rd Floor, Suite 3302
New York, NY 10005
USA

mail-usa@austinmacauley.com
+1 (646) 5125767

Acknowledgments usually imply gratitude. I have no gratitude for the Coronavirus pandemic, but the enforced inactivity that it imposed led me to put these long-pondered ideas into a coherent form.

I am, however, grateful for the help I received. In particular, I want to thank my friend, the psychotherapist, Edward Garcia, for his input regarding the psychological aspects of habits in the final two chapters.

And as always, my wife, Mary, was my best support, both by enduring the hours I spent at my keyboard and by proofreading (for the second time!) a book even though she had no reason to be interested in it. Love is wonderful!

Table of Contents

Preview	11
Introduction	12
Chapter 1: A Nation of Dieters	20
Chapter 2: You Are What You Eat	31
Chapter 3: Counting Calories	42
Chapter 4: How Diets Work – or Don't	50
Chapter 5: Burning Calories	62
Chapter 6: Exponential Weight Loss	69
Chapter 7: The Yo-Yo Diet Plan	78
Chapter 8: How to Weigh Less	86
Chapter 9: How Much Should You Weigh?	97
Chapter 10: Weight Loss that Lasts	110
Appendix A: The Mifflin-St Jeor Equation	121
Appendix B: The Calculus of Weight Loss	124
Appendix C: Diet Versus Exercise	127

Preview

It isn't hard to lose weight if you know how.

You don't need to starve yourself on diet meal plans with only a thousand calories a day – you can lose ten pounds or more by cutting out just a can of soda or a bag of potato chips. Exponential weight loss lets you weigh less and keep your weight where you want it – forever.

Every year, tens of millions of Americans spend tens of billions of dollars losing weight. But their average weight keeps climbing. Something clearly isn't working as it should.

This book explains why diets don't work and reveals the secret of weighing less on a long-term basis, based on a scientific understanding of why and how the weight of your body changes. It tells you the easy way to weigh less permanently, rather than doing the yo-yo – losing weight quickly and then regaining it, over and over again. And it shows that your health doesn't depend on being as thin as a stick.

Introduction

**"You are obese. You need to lose some weight,"
my doctor said.**

If you're like me, the thought of being "obese" is repugnant. When my physician used that word, I rebelled internally; surely I wasn't really "obese!" Maybe I was a few pounds heavier than when I was younger, but certainly I was not one of those people whose lack of self-discipline results in huge bellies hanging over their belts.

"Obese" is, after all, basically a *mean* word. Using it is the opposite of paying a compliment. It carries an image of people who not only are enormously fat but also can't control their appetites. That weakness is an occasion for shame. When House Speaker Nancy Pelosi called President Donald Trump "morbidly obese" in 2020, she was accused of "fat-shaming." Although the dictionary defines *obese* as "Grossly fat or overweight," to most of us it is a value judgment as well as a clinical description. Being obese is shameful.

But when I objected, my doctor gave me information from the Centers for Disease Control and Prevention (CDC), a part of our federal National Institutes of Health. It showed their official weight classifications based on something called the Body Mass Index (BMI). The BMI is obtained by dividing your weight in kilograms by the square of your height in meters (or equivalently, dividing your weight in pounds by the square of your height in inches and multiplying by 703.)

Based on the BMI, the CDC has categorized people in the following way:

BMI greater than 40:	"Severely or Morbidly Obese"
BMI between 30 and 40:	"Obese"
BMI between 25 and 30:	"Overweight"
BMI between 18.5 and 25:	"Normal or Healthy"
BMI less than 18.5:	"Underweight"

I had a BMI of 32.5, which meant that I was indeed "Obese" according to the CDC's labels. Donald Trump's BMI, based on his listed weight and height, was 30.5. He too was "Obese" – not "Morbidly Obese," as Nancy Pelosi called him, but certainly "Obese." Pelosi was not entirely wrong, but she wasn't the one who was "fat-shaming" Trump; the shaming came from the CDC, whose choice of the pejorative word "Obese" shamed everybody with a BMI over 30.

Was I really one of those shamefully fat people?

"Have you thought about joining Weight Watchers or trying one of the other diet plans?" my doctor suggested.

I knew about those plans. Like most Americans, I had tried them over the years, without lasting success.

I wasn't always fat. Up to the age of five or six, I was not a healthy kid, always sick with respiratory problems, and I had no appetite. I was so thin that my mother would not take me out wearing shorts – my skinny legs embarrassed her. But then I had my tonsils removed and my health improved drastically. I had an appetite, and my mother was so happy to see me gaining weight that she let me eat anything and everything I wanted. And I was proud of myself because I was making my mother happy, so I ate and ate. Within a year or two I was the second-heaviest kid in my second-grade class, second only to my pal Harry who was a real "ball of lard." He and I anchored the line on our fifth-grade football team. I was "fat and happy."

But a few years later I discovered girls, and I also discovered that they were generally not keen on fat boys. So I began my life-long pursuit of being thinner. Our daily newspaper carried a daily pseudo-psychology column written by a Dr. Crane. One of his columns pointed out that our bodies are over 50% water and suggested that I could lose weight simply by restricting my water intake. I eagerly tried going thirsty. Nothing much happened at first but finally, after a few days, I lost a pound!

Of course, when I quit dehydrating my body, it returned to its normal healthy fluid balance, and the weight returned. Prize fighters and jockeys have used this trick for years before weigh-in; they get a quick weight loss via dehydration, and then they get it back by restoring the lost fluid when the weigh-in is over. Dr. Crane's weight-loss trick worked, but only for a short time. The weight came back.

Since then, throughout my life, I have tried various weight-loss plans. I tried the Atkins plan* of cutting out carbohydrates. It worked; I lost several pounds over the next month. But it was hard to ask my wife to plan low-carb meals for me when she and my daughter weren't interested in losing weight and didn't need to be. Eventually, I couldn't ask them to suffer any further because of me, so I went back to our normal family meals.

And over the next few months, the weight came back.

I tried Weight Watchers. I paid my fee, ate what they told me to, went to meetings faithfully, reported how much I had lost. And a few pounds came off by the end of the six-week session. But, as with cutting out carbohydrates, I couldn't eat what I wanted, or what our family meals usually included. So I didn't sign up to continue attending and went back to normal eating.

And over the next few months, the weight came back.

The greatest success I had resulted from Dr. Kenneth Cooper's book *The New Aerobics*,* which introduced me to the benefits of running. I had never been an athlete, but when my colleagues at work began running after reading his book, I decided to give it a try. I started running several days each week with friends who generously put up with my initial struggles. Surprisingly, I liked it! And my weight

---

* *Dr. Atkins' Diet Revolution: The High Calorie Way to Stay Thin Forever.* D. McKay Co., 1972.
* *The New Aerobics*, Kenneth H. Cooper. New York, Bantam Books, 1970.

came down, slowly but steadily. The more I ran, the more I lost. I continued running for many years. Sometimes work issues would make me run less or even skip a month or two, and my weight would creep back up a bit; but when I got back to my routine, it went back down.

Eventually, though, life caught up with me. Back problems and extra responsibility at the office combined to restrict my running and finally to eliminate it entirely. I miss it to this day, but I reached a point where I just couldn't continue running.

And over the next couple of years, all the weight I had lost came back.

Insanity, they say, is doing the same thing over and over again and expecting different results. I was one of those insane people.

I am, by education, a physicist. With a Ph.D. from Cambridge University, I became a Professor of Physics at Iowa State University before yielding to the siren song of administration and becoming a dean and a vice-president. As a physicist, I published numerous papers analyzing data on quarks. That required me to understand how to create a mathematical description of things that were happening. After I saw that running led to weight loss, I applied some of those analytic methods to what was happening to my weight. I developed a mathematical model showing that running a mile a day, without increasing what you ate, would lead to a weight loss of about 5%.

And that prediction turned out to be true for me. Over the years, as my running mileage varied, my weight varied to follow it, in about the amounts my model suggested. When my wife took up running too, I predicted how much weight she would lose, and my prediction was correct. We both ran happily for many years, and weighed less while we did, until our aging bodies told us that if we wanted to still be walking comfortably in our eighties, it was time to give it up.

Since my model turned out to be valid for running, I continued to study the question of how exercise affects your weight. Some of my research, regarding energy optimization in swimming, got published in the scientific literature. A few years later I adapted my model to describe dieting instead of exercise. When I did, I found that the drastic calorie reduction required by commercially marketed diets is neither effective nor healthy – my model, based on over a century of nutritional research, revealed that a small reduction in calories is all it takes to lose a significant amount of weight.

You don't need to go on one of the popular diet plans that cut your calories by half or more. A *small* change in how much you eat and drink can result in a *big* weight loss. You can lose five to ten pounds just by giving up just a glass of wine, or a can of soda, or a bag of potato chips. That's hard to believe, but it's true. I know, because I did it.

This small reduction doesn't result in rapid weight loss. It's slow – it will take a couple of years to reach your target weight. You lose weight according to what scientists call an exponential decrease, which is why I call it *exponential weight loss*. But it's both effective and healthy. And it's much easier than trying to endure extremely low-calorie diets for a month or two and then fighting to keep the weight off.

That is the message that inspired this book.

Along the way, I learned that although tens of millions of Americans spend tens of billions of dollars each year on weight loss, they have not lost weight. Instead, they have gained steadily – over thirty pounds, on average, since 1962. The reason is simple: diets are inevitably temporary, and temporary diets cannot bring about permanent weight loss. Instead, after we diet and lose weight, we stop dieting and gain it back – the "yo-yo" diet syndrome that is both disheartening and unhealthy.

In the process, I also discovered that the CDC's description of your health status based on your BMI is seriously flawed. Contrary to their labels and warnings, the average American, who is supposedly "Overweight" and almost "Obese" with a BMI just under 30, is less likely to die of weight-related causes than those with BMI's below 25, whom the CDC considers "Normal or Healthy." In fact, if your BMI is between 20.7 and 29.8, your mortality risk resulting from weight puts you in the healthier half of the population.

I set my goal to lose enough weight to get into that healthy range via exponential weight loss, and I achieved a healthy, happy weight without continuously dieting and battling the scales. It required a change in my eating habits, but only a very small one. And I found out how to make that change easy.

In this book, I want to share what I discovered, so that you can do that too.

When you lose weight exponentially, your body follows its natural path to a new weight. You don't have to suffer through eating only the extremely-low-calorie meals required by some diet plan you saw on the web or television;

eat as you normally do, except for giving up an amount so small you probably won't even miss it. And you don't have to worry about gaining the weight back when the diet ends, because there's no diet to end.

I am going to show you how to really weigh less, rather than just losing weight temporarily and then regaining it. It requires a long-term change in what you eat and drink. That's the bad news. The good news is that it's such a small change you may not even notice it.

You can do that. I'll show you how.

Chapter 1
A Nation of Dieters

We have been a nation obsessed with dieting for many years. But it hasn't done us much good; in fact, we're less healthy now than we were.

Americans became weight-conscious long before the CDC labeled me "Obese." We have been counting calories since as early as 1887, when a series of articles appeared in a popular magazine called *Century*. The articles, by Wilbur O. Atwater, a nutrition researcher, described how the energy contained in food, measured in calories, was important to its nutritional value. Soon afterward, in 1894, the US Department of Agriculture published the first US tables showing the calorie content of various foods.

In the early 1900s, physician Lulu Hunt Peters published a series of newspaper columns followed by a best-selling book, "*Diet and Health: With Key to the Calories.*" That book made the general public aware, for the first time, of the relationship between calorie consumption and weight. Since then, we have been trying to lose weight by reducing the number of calories we take in daily. Almost every new decade has brought a new diet craze.

In the 1920s, the Lucky Strike cigarette brand suggested that people could "keep a slender figure" if they would "Reach for a LUCKY instead of a sweet," based on the belief that nicotine suppresses the appetite and consequently reduces calorie intake. And in fact, that is true; most people who quit smoking do gain from five to ten pounds. Part of this gain reflects the fact that nicotine increases your metabolism so that your body burns more calories. But it's also true that many people satisfy the unfulfilled nicotine craving by eating. So smoking does lead to weighing less, but we now know that it isn't a safe way to lose weight.

In the 1930s, the Grapefruit Diet became popular, first in Hollywood and then nationally, by promising that you could lose weight by eating grapefruit with every meal. Originally known as the "18-Day Diet," it claimed that grapefruit has "fat-burning enzymes," a claim that is still made even though research has found no evidence to support it. The diet did produce quick weight loss, but it had nothing to do with grapefruit; in addition to eating grapefruit, it required reducing your daily intake to about 800 calories, far below normal or healthy levels, for eighteen days.

In various altered forms, the Grapefruit Diet continues to be advertised in supermarket tabloids and online, promising. for example, that you can "lose 12 pounds in 10 days." As I'll show later, losing weight that rapidly is physically impossible. But that doesn't stop the marketers or deter those who fall for their ads.

In a very similar way, the Cabbage Soup Diet became a hit in the 1950s by proposing that including cabbage in every meal would result in a loss of 10-15 pounds in just a week. Like the Grapefruit Diet, it produced quick weight loss, not because of any magic ingredient in cabbage, but because it required an extreme reduction in calorie intake. And like the Grapefruit Diet, it is still around and still spouting the same silliness.

In 1963, dieting evolved from a craze to a business when Jean Nidetch, a housewife in Queens, New York, created the original Weight Watchers diet and program. Like many popular diets, it was based on eating lean meat, fish, skim milk, and fruits and vegetables, and it banned alcohol, sweets, and fatty foods. But it also combined food restrictions with a support program, which was a new idea that became the key to its huge success. In addition to providing a diet, the Weight Watchers plan relies on group psychology – you attend regular meetings at which you stand up and tell everyone how you're doing, which provides a powerful stimulus to stick to the diet.

Thanks to this innovation, Weight Watchers became immensely popular. Since its 1963 beginning, it has grown to the point that it regularly has over a million participants. It has even automated the weight loss process, thanks to a new app for your phone which "learns how you eat, move, sleep and think – because science shows it all matters when it comes to losing weight."

Other diet businesses followed, responding to the popular appeal and financial success of Weight Watchers. In 1972, Nutrisystem began to offer weight loss counseling and products in its own stores, competing directly with Weight Watchers; but in 1999, the company changed its business model and began selling pre-made low-calorie meals directly to consumers. Nutrisystem promises that by using its products you can "Lose up to 13 lbs & 7 inches overall in your first month!"

Similar programs relying primarily on selling ready-to-eat meals to their customers followed Nutrisystem's model. The Jenny Craig company began selling its brand of meals in Australia in 1983 and now does so worldwide; the South Beach Diet has done the same since 2003.

A different approach to losing weight appeared in 1972 when cardiologist Robert C. Atkins introduced the low-carbohydrate diet scheme. In his book he proposed that weight loss could be brought about by reducing your intake of carbohydrates, rather than cutting calories. The book's popularity led to commercialization, with a line of low-carb packaged foods widely available on supermarket shelves plus numerous cookbooks and other guides.

Losing weight by taking pills has also been a popular weight loss technique. In 1952, for example, "Dr. Parrish's Tasty Tablet Plan" promised that you could "LOSE UGLY FAT IN ONLY 7 DAYS" with "No Harmful Drugs! No Complicated Diets! No Need To Deny Yourself Delicious Foods!" The heart of the plan was that you would "eat 8 Dr. Parrish's Tasty Tablets" instead of lunch. Beyond that, you could "eat any food you like in sensibly reduced portions." Of course, it was those "sensibly reduced portions" that led to weight loss, whether or not the Tasty Tablets were involved.

Dr. Parrish's Tasty Tablets disappeared from the scene, but other pharmaceutical diet plans followed in their footsteps. Dexatrim promised in the 1980s that you could lose weight by using their pills, which combined the decongestant phenylpropanolamine with the amphetamine-like compound ephedra. Unfortunately, in addition to weight loss, phenylpropanolamine and ephedra were also linked to a higher incidence of strokes and heart problems, and the Food and Drug Administration (FDA) required Dexatrim to be removed from the market. A modified version remains available, but no claims of its efficacy and safety have been approved by the FDA.

A new drug combination called Fen-Phen met a similar fate in the late 1990s after it was found that its two primary ingredients, taken together, destroy the body's ability to control the amount of serotonin in blood plasma and that one of them, fenfluramine, was also linked to heart valve problems. The FDA, after initially approving it, responded when these risks became recognized and required Fen-Phen to be removed from the market.

The FDA regulates products like Dexatrim and PhenFen because they are considered medications. Supplements that can be sold over the counter, however, don't need FDA approval before they are marketed. As a result, the market is full of supplements promising weight loss, most or all of which are unverified and probably ineffective. For example, makers of chromium-based supplements claim that they can lower your appetite, help you burn more calories, reduce your body fat, and increase your muscle mass. But a review of 24 studies that checked the effects of 200 to 1,000 micrograms of chromium a day found no significant benefits.

Beyond being ineffective, these unregulated supplements can actually be harmful; the FDA discovered 72 over-the-counter weight loss products that could potentially compromise consumers' health. Among the ingredients in these 72 products were many unreported pharmaceuticals, some of which are known to have possible side effects including heart attacks, seizures, and strokes.

These are but a few of the plans that have marketed their magical methods of losing weight to the American public. Some of them do produce quick weight loss. Others produce primarily quick profit for the companies that sell them. Their advertising has persuaded the American public that it is important "to keep a slender figure," as Lucky Strike described it a century ago – that they need to weigh less than they do.

Their emphasis on losing weight took on a new urgency in 1998, when the CDC revised its BMI categories to conform to those applied worldwide by the World Health Organization even though there was no evidence that health norms elsewhere were the same. The new scale lowered the borderline between "Overweight" and "Normal or Healthy" from 27.8 to 25. a change that made over 29 million Americans who had previously been "Normal or Healthy" become "Overweight" and unhealthy overnight, although they had not gained an ounce.

Government and health agencies soon began emphasizing that excess weight was dangerous, issuing such warnings as:

"Obesity is epidemic in the United States today and a major cause of death." (CDC program)

"Obesity is a grave public health threat, more serious even than the opioid epidemic." (The Commonwealth Fund blog, April 24, 2018)

"If immediate action is not taken, millions will suffer from an array of serious health disorders." (World Health Organization website)

It really makes you think that fat people are dying by the dozens in the streets, doesn't it?

And the public responded to these panic-stricken warnings, coupled with aggressive advertising by the diet industry, by becoming a nation of obsessive dieters.

If you have succumbed to the CDC's warnings and tried to lose weight, you're far from alone. Americans have become addicted to dieting. According to the Washington Post, about 45 million Americans went on a diet in 2017. A report from the CDC found that 49% of American adults surveyed between 2013 and 2016 reported trying to lose weight at some point during the prior 12 months. Those whom the CDC labeled "Obese" were especially vulnerable to the CDC campaign; two-thirds of "Obese" adults had tried to lose weight. Although almost all of those who were labeled "Overweight" weighed less than the average adult, 49% of them dieted; they had been led to believe that their health, as well as their appeal to others, was at risk. And even one-fourth of those with "Normal or Healthy" BMI values were infected by the weight-loss push, although they were not considered by the CDC to be in any need of losing weight.

Diet plans are now big business, making a huge profit by selling you their products. Americans spent $72.7 billion on weight-loss products in 2018, and the amount is expected to continue growing at 2.6% annually. The leader is Weight Watchers, now known as WW International, Inc. Its income is based primarily on charging a subscription fee to participate in its meetings and online programs, although it also offers purchasable food products. These fees and other products generated annual revenues exceeding $1,500,000,000 in 2018.

Others, such as Nutrisystem, South Beach, and Jenny Craig, make big profits by selling you their pre-made meals. Nutrisystem was purchased by a company called Tivity Health, Inc. for $1.3 billion in 2018 and brings in revenues exceeding $600,000,000 per year. Jenny Craig began business in Australia in 1983; it is now owned by a Miami-based private equity firm called HIG Capital. Although its financial figures are not public, they are probably comparable to Nutrisystem's. The South Beach Diet business was initially very similar to Jenny Craig, and it has remained so since Nutrisystem acquired it in 2017. All three plans continue to offer pre-made low-calorie meals and make a profit when you buy them. That's why they are in business.

The Atkins plan became popular – and profitable – when the book's popularity led to its commercialization, with a line of low-carb packaged foods becoming available on supermarket shelves plus numerous cookbooks and other guides. After several permutations, the Atkins Diet Plan book and meals are now the property of a business imaginatively called "The Simply Good Foods Company." It has a current market capitalization over $1,600,000,000 based on annual revenues exceeding $650,000,000. Like the South Beach Diet, Jenny Craig, and Nutrisystem, it is now a big business, based on selling you its line of low-carb foods.

All these plans, and others like them, are part of an enormous weight-loss industry. In addition to the products they sell directly, they have spun off a multitude of books, magazines, and other subsidiary businesses. They make tens of billions of dollars in profits each year by catering to the public's desire to lose weight. They offer different ways to reduce calories – some sensible, some not – but if you follow them and reduce your calorie intake, you will probably lose some weight while you do.

And because people have come to believe that fat is inherently unhealthy and ugly, and that it's better to be thin, they continue to buy the products.

But have they worked?

Do people really weigh less?

You would think that the American public, responding to the CDC's warnings, would have used the methods offered by the weight-loss industry to create a leaner, healthier America. You would think that Americans would not spend over $72,000,000,000 annually on dieting without seeing successful, sustained weight loss. You would think that these diets would have worked. You would think that the average weight of the American public would have decreased.

In fact, just the opposite has occurred.

Despite the CDC's warnings and the overwhelming business success of the diet industry, the average American has gained weight steadily, as shown in Figure 1.

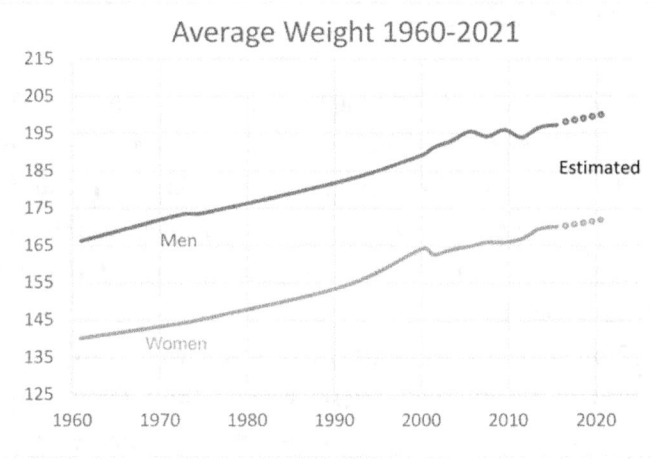

Figure 1. The growth of Americans' average weight since 1960 (data from https://www.cdc.gov/nchs/data/nhsr/nhsr122-508.pdf)

According to the CDC's latest published data, in 2015-16 the average American man weighed 197.3 pounds, and the average American woman weighed 170.1 pounds. Extrapolating to 2021 suggests an average weight of about 200 pounds for men and 172 pounds for women. That's a big gain – about 20% – since 1960–62, when the average man weighed only 166.3 pounds, while the average woman weighed 140.2 pounds.

That means our average weight has increased by over thirty pounds since 1962. Both men and women have gained, on average, more than half a pound per year for the last sixty years. Average height didn't change significantly during that period; we just got bigger around. Despite all the diet companies' ads and the CDC's warnings, we didn't lose weight – we gained it.

Clearly, something isn't working as expected. We have been spending billions of dollars on weight-loss products and millions of taxpayer dollars proclaiming that we're in a grave health crisis because of weight. Yet we have been gaining weight continuously. What are we doing wrong?

The answer is obvious: diets don't work. Despite the weight loss industry's promises and the CDC's panic-stricken warnings, Americans weigh more than ever and continue to gain. If we want to weigh less, a new solution is needed.

That solution is what this book is all about. In the next chapter, I'll tell you why we gain or lose weight.

Chapter 2
You Are What You Eat

There's truth in the old saying "You are what you eat." Everything in your body got there through your mouth, except what you were born with – and that came via your mother's mouth. The converse isn't true, of course – everything that comes in through your mouth doesn't stay in your body. You get rid of most of it. What you are is the difference between what you take in and what you get rid of. In this chapter I'm going to tell you why what you get rid of isn't the same as what you take in.

Albert Einstein is one of my heroes. He was passionately devoted to simplicity. "Everything should be as simple as possible," he said. Then he added, "But no simpler." To comprehend as simply as possible the contradiction between constant dieting and continuous weight gain, you have to begin by understanding what causes your weight to change. And that actually depends primarily on the two quantities Einstein most famously studied – mass and energy.

It's a basic law of physics that mass and energy are conserved – they can change form or location, but they never simply appear or disappear*. If you throw a ball up into the air, you change chemical potential energy stored in your muscles to the kinetic energy of the ball's motion and then to the potential energy of its height, but the amount of energy never changes. Potential energy changes to kinetic energy and then back to potential energy, but in precise amounts that maintain the same total. The conservation of energy is a basic truth of the universe, as made law by Newton. Energy can change forms, but the total amount never changes.

And the same is true for mass. The same total amount is always there; it never changes. If you start with a certain amount of mass, you can move it around, you can change its shape or even its chemical composition, but you can't change the total amount of mass.

Weight is a measure of mass interacting with gravity. As long as you're on the surface of the earth, gravity is essentially constant, and weight is directly proportional to mass. If the amount of mass never changes, neither does the amount of weight. Like mass, weight can change locations or shape or chemical composition, but it can't appear from nowhere, nor can it vanish.

If you hold an eight-ounce steak in your hand and step on the scales, the scales will show how much you and the steak together weigh, that is, your weight plus eight ounces

---

* You can, of course, convert mass to energy, as Einstein showed in his formula $E=mc^2$. Fortunately, that doesn't happen in our bodies, so it doesn't have anything to do with weight. If it did, the mass of an eight-ounce steak would provide the total daily calories used by 1.3 million people – a lot of energy!

for the steak. If you weigh 172 pounds without the steak, and the steak weighs half a pound, the scales will register 172.5 pounds.

If you eat that eight-ounce steak, having it in your stomach is the same as having it in your hand, as far as the scales are concerned; the steak may have disappeared from sight, but its weight is still pressing down on the scales through your feet. So after you have eaten it, the scales will still show 172.5 pounds. You will weigh eight ounces more with the steak in your stomach than you did when it was still in the refrigerator.

Similarly, if you drink eight ounces of water, you will then weigh eight ounces more than you did before you picked it up and drank it. And if you get rid of four ounces of urine, you will weigh four ounces less when you finish than you did before you started.

Whatever you put into yourself adds to your weight as soon as you consume it. Whatever you get rid of reduces your weight as soon as you get rid of it. It doesn't matter what it is, only how much it weighs. Whether you eat steak or drink water, if it weighs eight ounces, you gain eight ounces. Whatever you get rid of, if it weighs four ounces, you lose four ounces. At the end of the day, if what you got rid of didn't weigh the same amount as what you took in, your weight will change by the difference between the two.

Weight never disappears – it only changes location, when it goes from outside you to inside you or from inside you to outside you. When the amount that's inside you changes, your body's weight changes.

From a physics point of view, it's that simple. What isn't simple is why what you get rid of may weigh more or less than what you take in.

That involves some complex subjects. Nutrition is not simple – there are many factors affecting how much you eat, why you eat it, what your body needs, and why your body needs it. The human body, and its digestive processes, are not simple. How the stuff you eat and drink makes it possible for you to move your muscles involves complicated biochemistry.

Those are major fields of study, and they deal with complex issues. But while they are important to your health, they have little direct effect on your weight. All the nutritionists' concerns about getting enough of necessary vitamins and minerals and maintaining your chemical balance don't directly affect how much you weigh. Neither do the details of digestion or muscle activation.

Changes in your weight result from adding weight to your body or removing weight from your body. And you can understand that process without knowing the details of nutrition and digestion.

Most people think of their weight as a number that doesn't change rapidly. They get on the scales each morning to see whether they gained or lost since yesterday, and they don't weigh again until the next morning. Or they weigh at the doctor's office, when it's required, and don't think about it until the next visit.

But in fact, your weight is constantly changing, and by far more than you probably realize. You are adding stuff to your body and removing stuff from your body all the time, and as a result, your weight is changing all the time too.

Coordinated estimates of the average person's input and output – solid, liquid, and gas – are hard to find. Nobody seems to have looked systematically at the overall picture of how much weight we put into our mouths daily versus how much we get rid of. No data are available that directly compare your food and drink intake with your waste output, but the data that are available on these items separately suggest that the average American probably takes in six or seven pounds of food and drink per day and gets rid of about the same amount.

Of course, it doesn't all happen at once. The weight comes in and goes out at different times – people typically eat three meals a day, plus maybe some snacks; drink more often; defecate once; urinate maybe four or five times, some more, some less.

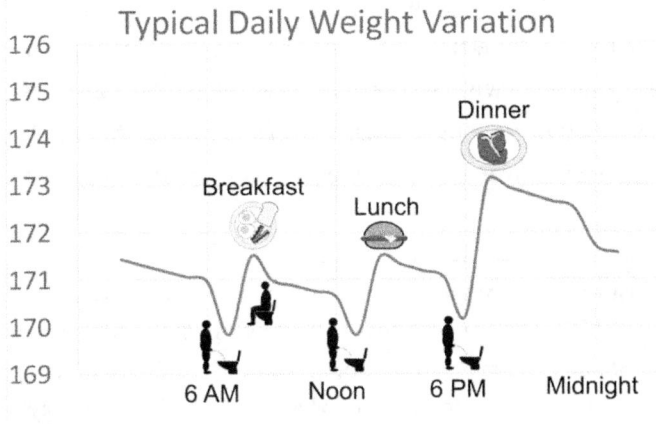

Figure 2. How your weight might vary during an average day

So your weight will vary throughout the day according to when you eat and drink, when you go to the bathroom, and a variety of other factors. If you track it, you'll find that during an average day your weight can easily vary by as much as three or four pounds, as shown in Figure 2.

If you are watching your weight, it's essential to weigh consistently at the same time each day. Your weight will probably be at its lowest after you urinate when you get up in the morning. Then you'll gain with each meal and snack, reaching your heaviest weight after dinner; and you'll lose with each urination and bowel movement, while you're also losing continuously via perspiration and respiration[*].

This is a simplified picture of the process, of course. Your intake of food and drink isn't the same every day, and neither is your digestion. Some days you eat more than other days; at Christmas dinner, for example, people may eat about twice as much as they usually do. So the day after Christmas, you will weigh more than you would have without all that extra turkey.

And over the next several days, you will weigh more than you otherwise would, because what you eat doesn't pass through you immediately. It takes food two or three days to pass through your digestive system. It doesn't all go

---

[*] Most of daily weight loss is liquid, via urine and perspiration; less than a pound is solid waste. But surprisingly, you actually lose about a pound and a quarter each day just by breathing, because the carbon dioxide you exhale is heavier than the oxygen it replaces in the air you inhale. If you weigh before going to bed and again when you get up the next morning, you'll see that you lost weight just by breathing and perspiring during the night.

through you at the same rate; liquids and sweets are probably gone the next day, but meat and roughage need four or five days to get through your digestive tract. If you eat that eight-ounce steak mentioned earlier, your weight will stay higher for four or five days, because the meat will take that much longer to make its way through your intestines. Similarly, the extra weight from the Christmas turkey will linger in your intestinal tract for several days and keep your weight higher than it would have been. That extra weight will ultimately pass on through your system, but you'll weigh more until it does.

A similar thing happens if you suddenly reduce your food intake. Most diets, whether they call for reducing calories or follow some other method, require you to eat significantly less food than previously. Nutrisystem, for example, offers five days' worth of meals in a box weighing just over two pounds – less than half the weight of the food you would normally consume. So for several days after you begin to diet, you will lose weight because there's less going into your intestines, while you are getting rid of the normal amount that was already there, leaving you with less weight in your digestive tract. This quick loss may encourage you to think the diet is already working, but it's only a short-term effect, just like the weight gain that results from the big meal.

Eventually, you will return to your usual six or seven pounds of food and drink per day, since neither Christmas dinners nor diets last forever. When you do, your digestive tract, and the amount of stuff in it, will return to where it started. And your weight will do the same.

Other factors can also lead to weight variation over several days. Too much salt in your diet can result in fluid retention. Women may retain fluids according to their menstrual cycle. Heavy exercise will increase perspiration significantly, leading to weight loss. Drinking alcohol, coffee, or using other diuretics will also cause fluid elimination and do the same.

But all these changes are temporary. They last a few days or weeks but then they disappear. They don't contribute to your long-term average weight – the number that is "how much you weigh" – which is what's important for your health and happiness.

It's when you consistently take in more than you get rid of that long-term weight gain sets in. That is what has been happening to the American public over the last half-century. They have taken in more weight, day after day, than they have gotten rid of. To understand why that happens requires knowing what your body does with what you eat and drink. And that is all based on energy.

Your body requires energy for you to live. Every time you move a muscle in your body, it uses energy. Some of those muscle movements are involuntary – your heart beating, for example, or your lungs filling and emptying. Others are voluntary, ranging from everyday things like getting out of bed or walking across the room to vigorous exercise like running five miles. Whether it's walking, or breathing, or your heart beating, or even just thinking – it's a process that uses energy. It takes a certain amount of energy just to do whatever you do on a normal day.

Where does that energy come from? You can't create energy. If you need it for your body, you have to get it from somewhere. You get the energy your body requires from food and drink. Everything you eat is a source of energy. That's why you eat it. You are genetically programmed to eat and drink in order to get the energy your body requires.

You can think of your body using energy in the same way your car does. Energy is stored in the chemicals in whatever you eat and drink, just as it is stored in the chemicals in crude oil. The process of digestion converts those chemicals into fuel that your body can use to power muscle movement, just as a refinery converts crude oil into gasoline. The muscles in your body, like the engine of an automobile, burn the fuel, which releases the stored chemical energy and converts it into the mechanical energy of motion. Your body gets rid of the waste products produced by burning the fuel via your excretory systems, just as your car does via its exhaust system.

The fuel your body uses, in simplest terms, is fat. Of course, most of what you eat and drink is not fat – it's other stuff such as proteins and carbohydrates. But your digestive process converts some of that stuff into chemicals that your muscles use as fuel. The details are complicated, but you can understand what's happening pretty satisfactorily if you just think of that fuel as fat. Your digestive system refines food and drinks into fat, your muscles burn fat to get energy, and your waste disposal system gets rid of the stuff that is produced when the fat is burned.

Most of us only fill the gas tank in the car when it's getting close to empty. We don't do that with our body's energy reservoir – we eat, typically, three times a day, breakfast, lunch, and dinner, plus maybe an occasional snack. It's as if you add gasoline to your car's tank several times each day, rather than waiting until the tank is nearly empty – you add fuel to your body by eating and drinking throughout the day, rather than waiting until your fat supply is low.

If you put more gasoline in your car's tank on a given day than you use during that day, the unused gasoline remains stored in your tank. Since gasoline weighs about six pounds per gallon, your car will weigh more at the end of the day than it did at the beginning, by six pounds for each gallon of extra gasoline in the tank. Conversely, if you use more gasoline than you put into the tank, the car will weigh less, because you used some of the gasoline you had stored there previously.

Your body works the same way. Each day, you take in energy via food and drink, and your body converts it to fuel in the form of fat. Your muscles then burn fat to power your body. If you produce more fat than you use as fuel, your body stores it, just as your car stores gasoline you add to the tank but don't use. So at the end of the day, if you did not use up all the fat your digestive system produced from food and drink, your body will store the excess fat, and you will weigh more than you did to start the day. If you burn more fat than your digestive system produced, your body gets it from fat stored in your "fat tank." Unlike your car, your body has no fixed fuel tank; the fat is stored in cells throughout your body, and the available storage can increase – your "fat tank" expands as needed, adding inches to your waist and elsewhere.

That's what happens to the stuff you take in. Your digestive system uses some of it to produce fat; the rest just passes on through you. Your muscles burn fat as fuel to provide the energy your body needs; the byproducts of burning it also pass on through you. If you produce more fat than you burn, your body stores what's left; if you burn more than you produce, your body dips into its stored fat to make up the difference. What changes your weight is the difference between the amount of fat you produce and the amount you use.

It's that simple. Take in more energy than you use, and you store it in fat. Use more energy than you take in, and you get it by burning stored fat. Energy never disappears – if you don't use it, your body stores it. And the amount of energy that your body has stored, in the form of fat, determines how much you weigh. All the biochemistry of digestion and muscle movement is in the details of how that happens.

But the bottom line – how much you weigh, and how your weight changes – is simply the result of how much fat you have stored in your body. And that is determined by the balance between the energy you take in as food and drink and the energy you use to power your daily activities.

In Chapter 3, I'll tell you about energy you take in, which is measured in calories – that word the diet companies love to use.

Chapter 3
Counting Calories

Your weight is determined by the balance between the energy you consume and the energy you use. That makes it essential to understand how much energy is involved in your body's daily activities. In this chapter I'm going to tell you how we measure the energy in what you take in, how much of it common foods contain, and how much the average person takes in daily.

Energy is measured in different ways. When it's used by electric appliances, energy is usually measured in kilowatt-hours; that's how your electricity bill is calculated. When it's used to measure power-plant production, it's measured in British thermal units, or Btu's. When it's used to describe the energy released by a nuclear explosion, it's measured in kilotons, the energy released by exploding a thousand tons of TNT.

When we talk about the energy in food and drink or the energy we use in daily activities, we measure it in calories. The number of calories in food or drink is a measure of the amount of energy stored in them. When diets refer to calories, they are really describing energy, because that's what calories are – units of energy. Calories, or kilowatt-hours, or Btu, or kilotons are just different ways to measure energy, in the same way that inches or meters or miles are different ways to measure distances.

How much energy is a calorie? Technically, a calorie is defined as the amount of energy required to heat one gram of water by one degree Celsius. That's how the term is used by scientists. But when it's used in the popular media to describe the energy content of food, the same word "calorie" is usually – although incorrectly – used to describe one thousand of those scientific calories, which is properly called a *kilo*calorie. Sometimes people call this quantity a "Calorie" with a capital C, or a "Food Calorie" or a "Nutritional Calorie," to clarify that they mean a kilocalorie, not a calorie. But most publications and websites ignore the distinction and use "calorie" where they really mean "kilocalorie."

I'm going to do the same. So when I write "calorie" hereafter, I really mean *kilo*calorie, which is the amount of energy required to heat one kilogram of water by one degree Celsius – or, in US units, 2.2 pounds of water by 1.8 degrees Fahrenheit. A kilowatt hour is about the same as 860 of these calories; a kiloton is about a billion.

That's kind of hard to visualize, so let me give some examples:

- One calorie will keep a 60-watt bulb burning for a minute and ten seconds.
- A weightlifter will use about one calorie to lift 440 pounds from the floor to high above his head.

- A new AAA battery contains about 1.6 calories of stored energy; a 12.7-volt automobile battery has about 600.
- A 3000-pound car moving at 55 miles per hour has about 100 calories of kinetic energy.

It's relatively easy to know how many calories you take in each day. Since 1990, food labels have been required to list that information, which can be measured in the laboratory. So all you have to do is add up the calories in what you eat. The World-Wide Web is full of tables of the energy content of various foods and drinks. Table I gives a representative sample.

As you can see, the energy content of foods varies widely. The calories in a raw tomato will light up a 60-watt bulb for less than half an hour, while a double cheeseburger will keep it burning for almost half a day. The calories in a slice of pizza will let a weightlifter lift 440 pounds above her head more than 300 times. Accelerating your car to 55 mph takes the same amount of energy contained in a shot of whiskey.

The calorie content of food and drink relative to its weight also varies widely, from less than 100 calories per pound for lettuce to over 2700 calories per pound for nuts. The typical daily diet probably averages somewhere around 600 calories per pound. So if you enjoyed an extra six pounds of Christmas dinner, you probably took in an extra 3600 calories.

Item	Serving size	Calories
Apple, raw, with skin	6 ounces	90
Bacon	2 slices	70
Beer	12-ounce can	145
Cereal	1 cup	110
Chicken breast	3-ounce cutlet	142
Chocolate cake	4-ounce slice	642
Chocolate cookie	1.7 ounces	53
Cottage cheese, regular	1 cup	216
Double cheeseburger	7.6 ounces	550
Egg, scrambled	1 large	102
French fries	4 ounces	354
Ham, cooked	1 slice	46
Ice cream	1 cup	267
Lettuce	1 cup	8
Macaroni and cheese	1 cup	207
Milk	8 ounces	146
Mixed nuts	1 ounce	175
Orange juice	8 ounces	110
Pepperoni pizza	4-ounce slice	313
Pork chop, broiled	8 ounces	523
Potato chips, plain	1 ounce	155
Soda	12-ounce can	157
Steak, sirloin	5 ounces	344
Toast with butter and jam	1 slice	125
Tomato, raw	5 ounces	23
Whiskey	1.5-ounce glass	105
Wine, red or white	5-ounce glass	123

Table I: Calorie content of various foods

The CDC recommends that a healthy diet should provide between 1,600 to 2,400 calories per day for adult women and 2,000 to 3,000 calories per day for adult men. But the actual average daily calorie intake for Americans has long been considerably higher than that, as shown in Figure 3; it rose rapidly from 2861 in 1962 to 3833 in 2005, then declined about 5% through 2011. No new data have become available since 2011, but extrapolating from the data for 2005 through 2011 suggests a value[*] of about 3585 in 2020. That overall average corresponds to about 4010 calories per day for men and 3345 for women.

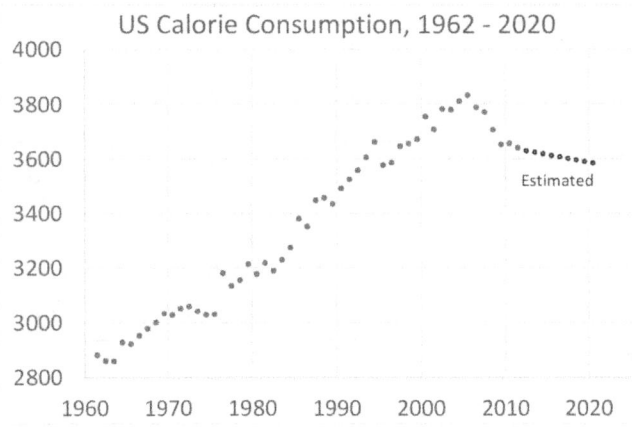

Figure 3. Americans' average calorie consumption since 1960 (Data from www.nationalgeographic.com/what-the-world-eats)

---

[*] Most of the figures in this book are approximate because of both roundoff in the calculations and statistical uncertainties in the data. But they are good approximations – they provide qualitative agreement with the actual results and a valid description of the outcomes.

Research has shown that the source of the calories doesn't matter at all, as far as your weight is concerned. An ounce of cereal is very different from eight ounces of orange juice, but the 110 calories contained in the cereal are identical to the 110 calories contained in the orange juice. Whether calories come from orange juice or from cereal, from a steak or from a beer, from lettuce or from peanuts, they are, simply, calories – the source is irrelevant.

The point was illustrated vividly by the so-called "Twinkie diet," in which Mark Haub, a professor of human nutrition at Kansas State University, ate almost nothing but "junk food" for 10 weeks. Every three hours, instead of a meal, he ate a Twinkie, or a few Oreos or potato chips, or some other form of junk food. Two-thirds of his total intake came from junk food. The other third came from vegetables and a daily protein shake, and he also took a multivitamin pill to help him maintain good health. On this "Twinkie diet," he lost 27 pounds.

Clearly, it doesn't matter what you eat – all that matters is how many calories you consume. If you consume more calories than your body uses, your body will store the excess energy in fat cells. If you consume fewer, your body will remove some fat from your fat cells and burn it to get the missing calories. It's this fat that is involved when you gain or lose weight.

Fat is not the largest part of your total weight – muscle and blood and skin and bones and various other tissues make up most of it. But there's a lot of fat. The average woman has about 40% of her total body weight in the form of fat; the average man has a smaller amount, about 29%. Fat is less dense than muscle or bone, so women, having more fat, are less dense than men; that's why they float more easily in the swimming pool.

Some of this fat – about 15 pounds for women, somewhat less for men – is essential for things like protective cushioning and insulation of vital organs. The rest – the fuel tank of energy described above – is stored, primarily subcutaneously, just under your skin. That's the amount that varies as you gain or lose weight. Based on the percentages given above, your body likely contains sixty or seventy pounds of fat, the energy equivalent of about fifteen hundred cans of soda.

The fat in your body contains about 3500 calories per pound. Taking in the American average of 3585 calories each day means creating a tiny bit more than a pound of fat to be used by your muscles or, if there's some to spare, stored in your body. It's about the same rate of energy production required to keep three 60-watt bulbs burning continuously, or to lift 440 pounds from the floor to up above your head every 24 seconds. You may be only about three times as bright as a 60-watt bulb, but there is still a lot of energy involved in your daily living.

You can think of your body as a fat factory. Each day you take in enough energy to produce about a pound of fat. And you burn about a pound of fat to power your body. When those two are in balance, your weight is stable. When they aren't in balance, your body winds up with more or less stored fat, and you gain or lose weight. Commercial diet companies get rich by persuading you to drastically upset that balance by severely reducing how much energy you take in daily. In the next chapter,

I'll show you how much weight loss they actually produce, which for many is less than they promise.

Chapter 4
How Diets Work – or Don't

If you want to diet, there are thousands of plans to choose from. In this chapter, I'm going to examine some of these plans in detail, and show you how much weight you can actually expect to lose by following them. Then I'm going to tell you why any of them is ultimately going to fail.

The list of commercial diet plans is almost endless. In fact, it may be endless – it was estimated that more than a thousand weight loss schemes had been developed by 2014, and new ones are being invented continuously. Besides the ones I've already described, you could choose the Military Diet, the GM Diet, the Paleo Diet, the Vegan Diet, the Zone Diet, or the Celery Juice Diet. You could even choose the Werewolf Diet, which limits what you eat based on the phases of the moon.

Most of these commercial diet plans restrict what you can eat. Some provide you with low-calorie meals to replace your normal menu, like Nutrisystem's. Others let you mostly choose for yourself, except that you must cut out some part of what you ordinarily eat – for example, the

Atkins plan lets you eat whatever you want, except that you have to avoid carbohydrates.

Either way, they lead to a severe reduction in your calorie intake which results in quick weight loss. By calculating how many calories they allow you, based on the quantitative understanding of energy developed in Chapter 3, it's easy to determine how much weight you will actually lose if you follow them.

Since the CDC found that women were more likely than men to report trying to lose weight, I'm going to talk about these plans as they would apply to an average American woman – one who weighs the average amount, 172 pounds, and takes in the average amount, 3345 calories daily. I'm going to call her Norma, because her weight and calorie intake are "normal," and calculate how much weight she would lose on each of several different diets. For an average man, similar calculations would lead to similar results.

If Norma is using 3345 calories daily, but she goes on a diet that provides fewer than that, she will need to burn enough stored fat to make up the difference. The amount of weight she will lose is easy to determine: she will lose a pound for every 3500 calories worth of stored fat she burns. For example, if she reduces her calorie intake by 1750 calories – a typical amount for commercial diets – that's one-half the calorie content of a pound of fat, so she will burn half a pound of fat daily.

Diet advertisements usually predict how much weight you will lose by following their plan. Some make a promise they can't keep – they promise that you will lose more than it's physically possible to lose. For an extreme example, the Military Diet (it has nothing to do with the US military but hopes you will think so) tells you that you can "Lose 10 pounds in 3 Days" by eating only what's on their diet plan. The sample meals they show for those three days total 3700 calories, an average of 1233 calories per day.

Consuming 3345 calories per day while taking in only 1233 calories means Norma needs to burn 2112 calories' worth of stored fat per day. Since a pound of stored fat can provide 3500 calories, she would need to burn about six-tenths of a pound – about 10 ounces – of fat per day in order to cover that energy shortfall. Over the three days, she would lose 1.8 pounds – not even two pounds, and certainly not ten.

Claiming that someone can lose ten pounds of stored fat in three days is preposterous. Since the energy content of a pound of fat is 3500 calories, losing ten pounds in three days would require a total calorie reduction of 35,000 calories, or 11,667 calories per day. But that average person isn't taking in anywhere near that many calories per day. You can't reduce your daily calorie intake by more than you're taking in. As I'll show in Chapter 5, taking in 11,667 calories per day would mean weighing six or seven hundred pounds. If you weigh less than that, you can't be taking in 11,667 calories daily, so there's no way to reduce it by that much.

Even taking in nothing at all – total starvation, zero calories – you won't burn that much stored fat. You might lose some weight temporarily as your digestive system empties, but you'll regain that amount when it refills, so that's not real weight loss. The most you can really lose is one pound for every 3500 calories.

So it's physically impossible to burn ten pounds of stored fat in three days. What they promise is simply not possible. Their ad is, to put it bluntly, a lie.

Many other diets promise faster weight loss than is physically possible. For example, a headline on the cover of "Woman's World," a supermarket aisle tabloid magazine, proclaimed on the cover of their February 24, 2020 issue that the "Best Detox Soup" would lead to a weight loss of 12 pounds in a week. At 3500 calories per pound of fat, losing 12 pounds in a week means burning 42000 calories worth of fat in seven days, an average of 6000 calories per day. As with the Military Diet, that's physically impossible. There's no reason to save the recipe for the soup.

Why does Woman's World publish such nonsense? It's all about the money. The front-page headline that says "Make one pot to lose 12 lbs this week!" is sucker bait. It seduces the gullible into buying the magazine, which is how they make a profit.

The South Beach Diet plan is similar, promising that Norma can lose "up to 7 lbs in your first 7 days" by eating only their pre-packaged meals. That would mean reducing your calorie intake by 3500 calories per day for seven days, more than the average American woman takes in daily. So, like the diets described above, it promises the impossible – Norma can't lose that much even if she eats nothing at all. But on the South Beach diet, she isn't eating nothing at all – the meal plans described on their website provide breakfasts, lunches, dinners, and snacks ranging between 100 and 300 calories each. Putting those together in a reasonable way, Norma would probably be consuming about 1000 calories per day, more or less.

So the South Beach Diet will actually mean a calorie reduction of around 2345 calories per day – far less than the 3500 calories it would take to lose a pound! She would actually be losing about 4.7 pounds per week rather than the promised seven pounds.

Their advertisement isn't quite a lie – they say you will lose "up to 7 pounds," which leaves open the possibility that you might lose less. You might only lose half an ounce, but that doesn't contradict their promise – they only said you will lose somewhere between zero and seven pounds. That's a standard advertising trick, including weasel words that allow the statement to seem stronger than it actually is.

As you can see, diet plans which advertise that you can lose a pound a day or more – or even "up to" a pound a day – should not be taken seriously. For most people, it simply isn't possible to burn that much fat.

There are, of course, diet plans that don't try to attract you with such outlandish come-on promises. Both Nutrisystem's plan and the Jenny Craig plan provide pre-made meals with about 1000 calories per day, very similar to those of the South Beach Diet. But Nutrisystem only teases that you can "lose up to 13 lbs" in a month, or 3 pounds per week; Jenny Craig only promises that you will lose "up to 16 lbs in your first four weeks," or 4 pounds per week. These loss rates would only require Norma to decrease her daily calorie intake by about half, so their ads are more credible.

Weight Watchers, as mentioned earlier, doesn't require you to buy pre-made meals. Neither do they count calories

– instead, they assign "points" to foods and give you a daily point target that will let you lose weight at a pound or two per week. The points are not identical with calories, but they are closely correlated; low-calorie foods such as vegetables get few or even zero points, while high-calorie foods full of sugar and fat get lots of points. While an apple gets zero points, a slice of apple pie gets 12 points. Basically, however, a Weight Watchers point is equivalent to about 50 calories, so counting points is really not significantly different from counting calories, just somewhat easier.

For an average woman like Norma, what would Weight Watchers accomplish? She would likely be assigned about 35 points per day, corresponding to roughly 1750 calories – more than the pre-made meal plans described above, but still significantly fewer than her normal 3345. Consequently, her weight loss would be slower and take longer than with Nutrisystem or Jenny Craig; she would burn about 1595 calories worth of fat each day and lose just over three pounds per week.

There are other plans that don't focus specifically on restricting your calories. Instead, they limit the kinds of things you can eat. If you have to leave out something you usually eat, you most likely will eat less. They get you to limit your total calorie intake by preventing you from eating some or all of what you normally eat. That leads you to eat less, so you reduce your calorie intake.

The most famous of these is the Atkins diet mentioned in Chapter 1. The current Atkins diet plan is similar to Nutrisystem and South Beach in that it is heavily invested in selling you their diet food products, but it is different in its approach to weight loss. This plan is based on the idea that most body fat results from eating carbohydrates, which are more easily converted to body fat than proteins or unsaturated fat.

Carbohydrates are a type of nutrient found in many foods and beverages. They occur naturally in many forms, including plant-based foods, such as grains; sugar is a carbohydrate often added to processed foods. The Mayo Clinic's *Dietary Guidelines for Americans* recommends that carbohydrates make up 45% to 65% of your total daily calories. It's reasonable to assume that most Americans fall into that range, so let's use the average figure of 55%.

The Atkins system suggests that you can eat as much protein and unsaturated fat as you want; as long as you avoid foods high in carbohydrates, they predict that you will still lose weight. How would that work for Norma? If 55% of her calories come from carbohydrates, she would be consuming about 1840 calories worth of carbohydrates daily.

The Atkins diet plan wants her to reduce her carbohydrate intake to 80 calories' worth. If she cuts out that many carbs and doesn't replace them with something else, such as protein or unsaturated fat, she will reduce her daily calorie intake by 1760 calories. A reduction of 1760 calories per day would result in losing about 3.5 pounds per week. The Atkins plan suggests, however, that she could eat more of other stuff and still lose weight by reducing her carbohydrates. But as shown in Chapter 3, what she eats doesn't matter – only the total calories it contains. If she cuts out 1760 calories worth of carbohydrates, but eats enough other stuff to maintain her normal 3345 calories per day, she won't lose an ounce. So what the Atkins plan really accomplishes is helping you find a healthy way to take in fewer calories.

Other diets work similarly, trying to get you to reduce your calorie intake by limiting your choice of food. There are low-fat diets that let you eat more other stuff but less fat, and high-fat diets that let you eat more fats but less other stuff. Probably the silliest of them is the GM Diet, which, like the Military Diet, wants you to believe that it originated in a trusted organization. It was supposedly created for the employees of General Motors in 1985 with help from the US Department of Agriculture and the FDA and extensive testing at the Johns Hopkins Research Center. But there is no evidence that any of this is true. Its true origins remain unknown. (That alone should make you suspicious!)

The GM diet claims to be "a panacea for all your weight loss needs" that, according to its website, will let you "Loose (sic) up to 17 pounds and even more in a week." You are supposed to accomplish that by eating only particular foods or food groups during each day of the diet. For example, on day 1 you are allowed to eat only fruits, and on day 2 of the diet, you can eat nothing but vegetables. The amount you can eat on each day is unlimited except that it must be in that day's category.

But as I've already shown, it's impossible to lose 17 pounds in a week – that would require a calorie reduction of 8500 calories per day, far beyond the calorie intake of almost anybody. And whether Norma eats only fruit is completely beside the point. If she eats, say, 5018 calories worth of strawberries, and nothing else, during Day 1, she won't "loose" an ounce – she'll gain half a pound!

Of course, Norma probably doesn't want to eat 5018 calories worth of strawberries or any other fruit. She probably doesn't even want to get her normal 3345 calories from only fruit and nothing else, in a day. If all she can eat is fruit, she will likely eat less in total than she usually does, and consequently consume fewer calories than her usual 3345. As a result, she will indeed lose some weight – but nowhere near 17 pounds in a week.

I guess you shouldn't expect much from an outfit that doesn't know the difference between "lose" and "loose"!

With any of these commercial diets, you lose weight rapidly because you reduce your calorie intake severely. That quick success is one of their selling points. But rapid weight loss creates physical problems for your body. Possible serious risks include gallstones, which occur in 12% to 25% of people who lose large amounts of weight on extremely low-calorie diets, and electrolyte imbalances, which can be life-threatening.

The greatest risk, however, is malnutrition. Diets achieving rapid weight loss don't provide the minimum number of calories Norma's body needs.

As mentioned in Chapter 3, the average American woman has about 40% of her body weight as fat; the average American man has about 29%. That means Norma, weighing 172 pounds when she starts dieting, has about 69 pounds of fat. Of this, about 54 pounds is stored subcutaneously as fuel for her daily activities; the remaining 15 pounds of fat is what's essential for life-critical tasks such as cushioning and insulating her body structure.

When Norma diets, she can lose the subcutaneous stored fat, but she needs to keep the 15 pounds of fat that's essential for her body to function. So the most she can lose and remain healthy is about 54 pounds. If she loses more than 54 pounds, she will begin to use up fat that her body needs for other purposes. If she is of average height and age, the least she can weigh and be healthy is about 118 pounds. Weighing less means becoming malnourished.

But on any of these extreme calorie reduction diets, she will lose 54 pounds within a few months. At that point, she must stop dieting or she will become malnourished. So even if these diets result in losing weight, they can't continue forever; eventually they must end.

And when the diet ends, the real problem begins. Norma may lose 13 pounds in a month with Weight Watchers or Nutrisystem or Atkins, but what will she do then? If she's like the millions of Americans who have dieted unsuccessfully, she will gain back every pound she lost, and maybe more.

That failure to maintain weight loss is common to most dieters. Many studies have shown that most dieters do not maintain their new weights. Typically, they regain 30% to 65% of the lost weight within one year. Within three years, 97% regain everything they lost, often more; one in three will end up heavier than they were before they dieted.

Regaining weight happens for several reasons. Under normal circumstances, your stored fat releases a hormone called leptin into the bloodstream. This hormone tells your brain when you have stored enough fat, making you feel full and stop eating. When you're dieting, having less fat in your body leads to decreased levels of leptin output. But when you stop dieting, you have less fat, so the leptin output doesn't fully return to its earlier pre-diet level. Because of that, your appetite increases. The result is that you eat more post-diet than you ate before you started dieting, and your weight goes up.

Dieting also forces you into a different and unpleasant lifestyle. That is stressful, and when you are stressed, your body secretes a hormone called cortisol. Cortisol stimulates your appetite, which makes it harder to lose weight and easier to gain it back.

Also, many studies have shown that when you lose weight on a very low-calorie diet, you lose muscle as well as fat. Cortisol is thought to be one of the causes of this loss. When the diet ends and you begin to regain the weight you lost, you regain fat first as your body stores the extra energy; rebuilding lost muscle tissue is a different, and much slower, process. As a result, when you get back up to your initial weight, you have more fat and less muscle than when you started. But your body still wants to replace the lost muscle, so your appetite stays in high gear and you wind up with as much muscle as you started with, and more fat.

The problem, then, is not that commercial diet plans don't result in weight loss; they do, in the extreme. But because they are extreme, they are necessarily temporary. And when they end, they have sown the seeds of their own failure, by making it almost unavoidable to regain the lost weight and likely more. That's why, as I pointed out in Chapter 2, the average weight of Americans keeps going up in spite of constant dieting.

The weight-loss business offers you thousands of ways to lose weight. The worst of them promise physically impossible results; the most effective of them

can produce weight loss of around three pounds per week. But these diets don't lead to permanent weight loss; regaining the lost weight is almost inevitable because most people take in more calories than they use when the diet is over. To understand how to avoid this failure, we need to find out more about the calories the body uses. In the next chapter, I'll tell you about that more complicated topic.

Chapter 5
Burning Calories

Knowing how many calories you use is much more difficult than knowing how many you take in. But it's the other half of the equation; comparing how much energy you use with how much energy you produce is the key to understanding why you gain or lose weight. In this chapter I'm going to introduce you to the science of metabolism.

The important thing to know is that the number of calories your body uses each day depends on your weight. If you think about it, that isn't surprising; it takes more force to move a heavier car than a lighter one, which means it must use more fuel to produce more energy. In the same way, it takes more energy to move the muscles that propel a heavier human body than a light one.

Scientists have studied how many calories people use daily. To properly describe their findings, I'll need to include a couple of equations. You can skip the equations and still understand the text; or if your eyes glaze over when you see an equation, you can skip to the end of this chapter, where the results are summarized. But if you'd like to understand more about how your metabolism works, read on.

You might expect that the energy used daily varies from person to person, and that is certainly true. Men use more energy per pound than women, for example, primarily because their bodies are denser with muscle. Older people use less energy per pound than younger people for the same reason, because they lose muscle as they age. The exact amount varies from individual to individual; it varies with gender, age, height, and activity level. Nutrition experts have nevertheless been able to develop ways of measuring the amount of energy required by average people.

The number of calories you use daily, called your Total Energy Expenditure (TEE), can be divided into three components. The most important, for sustaining your life, is the energy required by basic metabolic activities – maintaining your body temperature, breathing, powering vital organs such as the brain and the heart. This amount, called your Resting Energy Expenditure[*] (REE), typically accounts for about half of the average person's total energy expenditure.

The processes involved in digestion use about another 10% of the total, called the Thermic Effect of Food (TEF); they are also essential since they provide your body's energy requirements by converting what you eat and drink into your fuel supply.

The remainder of your energy usage powers the rest of whatever you do – the voluntary activities that make up your daily routine – and is called the Activity Energy

---

[*] Also called your Basal Metabolic Rate (BMR).

Expenditure (AEE). The AEE accounts for about 40% of the total for people with normal daily activities, but it can be a much larger portion for highly active folks like athletes, or much less for the elderly or infirm.

These three quantities make up the total amount of energy used by the body. Researchers have studied them, particularly the REE, in order to understand the human metabolism.

To find the REE, scientists studied people who were kept completely at rest in a neutral environment requiring neither heating nor cooling, so that no energy was used for any purposes other than the basic bodily functions. They determined the energy these subjects used – their REE – by carefully measuring the heat produced by their bodies. The most recent of these studies, carried out by Mifflin, St Jeor, and colleagues in 1990, determined the Resting Energy Expenditure of 498 healthy subjects, including 247 women and 251 men, of varying ages, heights, and weights. This study has become the standard reference on the subject (although, after thirty years, it probably needs to be updated.)

The details of their findings are given in Appendix A, for those who are interested; I'll just summarize what they learned. Their measurements showed that the Resting Energy Expenditure consists of four parts, each of which is proportional to one of four body characteristics – weight, height, age, and gender. These parts are independent of each other – the amount that depends on your weight doesn't depend on age, height, or gender, and so on. Adding these four components together yielded an equation that gave accurate values for the REEs of this representative group of people.

This research measured the Resting Energy Expenditure only, however – not the Total Energy Expenditure. To determine the TEE requires also knowing the Thermic Effect of Food and the Activity Energy Expenditure. The Thermic Effect of Food can be determined in a very similar way to the REE, by measuring the heat given off by people after they have eaten. But how do we account for the AEE, the energy used in all the other things we do? Clearly, that would be difficult to measure in the first place, and it would vary significantly from one person to another as well.

The Mifflin group suggested that in order to determine normal Total Energy Expenditure, the REE results should be increased overall by an "activity factor" to account for the rest of your daily energy usage. But as shown in Appendix A, that approach doesn't work very well. Instead, the Thermic Effect of Food should logically be assumed to be proportional to the number of calories being digested. And it is known that the energy used in most exercises – running or swimming, for example – is closely proportional to weight; there is little dependence on height, age, or gender. This suggests that the overall Activity Energy Expenditure should depend primarily on weight.

With these assumptions about the TEF and AEE, the total energy consumption TEE can be determined from the REE. The calculation is described in detail in Appendix A and leads to an equation for the Total Energy Expenditure given by

$$TEE = 15.3w + 17.7h - 5.47a + x$$

where w = weight in pounds, h = height in inches, a = age in years, and X is a factor depending on gender, given by x = -179 for women and x = +5.56 for men.

Is this formula correct? For any given individual, it's probably not exact – your TEE will depend on your body and your lifestyle, so the numbers in the equation will not be the same for everyone. But your TEE will depend on your weight, height, age, and gender in a way that is very similar to the above formula, and the proportionality to each of those factors will be somewhere close to that described by the formula. Whether it's exactly 15.3 times your weight doesn't matter so much; what matters is that it's somewhere near that value. It isn't as small as, say, 0.3, or as large as 89; it's somewhere close to 15.3, maybe 14.8 or 16.1 or something like that. In what follows, I'll use 15.3 calories per pound as a good average figure; the results may be off a bit for you if your body generates a different value, but it won't differ from 15.3 by much.

For people of average height who are 45 years old (the average age of the subjects used in the Mifflin study) this equation simplifies to

$$TEE = 15.3w + 714 \text{ for women}$$
$$TEE = 15.3w + 977 \text{ for men}$$

These two formulas provide a good approximation to the amount of energy an average American woman or man will use daily – about 15.3 calories per day to support each pound of weight, plus about 714 calories for women or 977 calories for men for other aspects of daily life.

What's important in this formula is how the number of calories you use daily depends on your weight. It also depends on your height and age; but your height and your age change too slowly to affect daily weight changes. So this first term, 15.3 times your weight, is the one that matters regarding diets and weight loss.

And it's significant – and perhaps surprising – that you only burn only about fifteen calories for each pound of weight. If you reduce your daily calorie intake by 15.3 calories, you won't be in balance; the weight your food intake can support is reduced by a pound, so your body will adjust by losing a pound. If you want to lose ten pounds, you only need to reduce your daily intake by 153 calories. That's a very small amount, compared to the calories you take in daily; since a pound of fat contains 3500 calories, you're making your body burn less than an ounce of stored fat per day. Your weight loss will be slow; but it will be sure, and far healthier than with the extreme reductions required by commercial diets.

Unfortunately, the opposite is also true – if your calorie intake exceeds your calorie usage by 15.3 calories, your body will be out of balance in the opposite direction, and it will respond by gaining a pound. If your calorie intake is 153 calories greater than the calories you use according to the TEE formula, you will gain ten pounds. That's why a short-term diet leads only to short-term results; if you go back to eating as you did before, your body will go back to weighing what it weighed before.

What scientific research has revealed, then, is that your energy usage is determined by your weight, as

described by the TEE formula, and that each pound of weight uses about 15.3 calories daily – a surprisingly small number. Since your weight will change if your calorie intake doesn't match your calorie usage, that means a small intake change – about fifteen calories – will lead to a one-pound weight change. You don't need to cut out thousands of calories with a painful commercial diet; cutting out about 150 calories, the amount in a can of soda, will yield a loss of ten pounds. But it also means your daily loss will be small, so it will take a lot longer to reach your goal. The entire process is different from what happens with commercial diets. In the next chapter, I'll examine how this works in more detail.

Chapter 6
Exponential Weight Loss

It's easy to calculate the total amount of weight you will lose from a diet. Dividing your daily calorie reduction by the 3500 calories in a pound of fat, as I did in Chapter 4, will tell you that amount. But if your daily calorie reduction is small, as suggested in Chapter 5, it will take a lot longer to lose the weight than on commercial diets. You'll need to persevere, and that's easier if you understand what's going on. In this chapter, I'll show you in more detail how much you can lose and how long it will take.

To illustrate how weight loss depends on the results of the previous chapter, let's start by supposing that our average woman Norma decides that she wants to lose 22 pounds, getting her weight down from 172 pounds to 150. She plans to accomplish that by losing a pound per week for 22 weeks. To make that happen, she needs to reduce her weekly calorie intake by the number of calories in a pound of fat – 3500 calories – which means a reduction of 500 calories per day. So she reviews her daily diet and alters it, in a way she feels she can comfortably maintain, to reduce her daily calorie intake by that amount.

A 500-calorie reduction isn't too difficult to live with, and she makes good progress at first. But then there's a problem, as shown in Figure 4. After the first few weeks, Norma notices that she's falling behind schedule. By the time three months have passed, she's more than two pounds above where she thought she would be. As days go by, the discrepancy gets worse. After the allotted 22 weeks, she weighs 156 pounds, rather than 150 as she expected.

So she keeps dieting. Finally, after almost 37 weeks, she reaches her goal of 150 pounds.

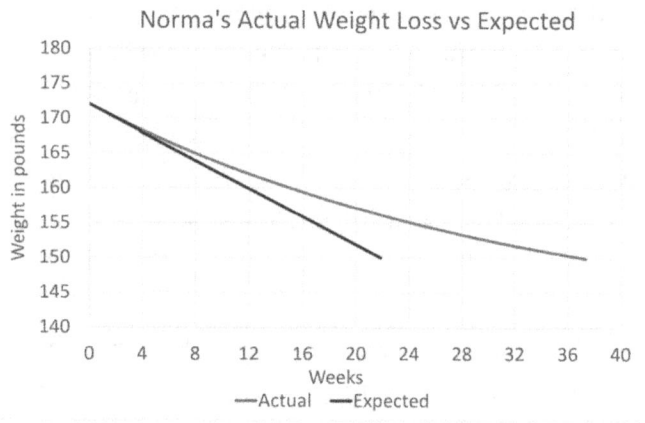

Figure 4. Norma's weight loss on 2845 calories daily

Why did it take her almost 37 weeks to lose 22 pounds, rather than 22 weeks as she expected?

Here's the reason. As she lost weight, her body needed fewer calories every day, according to the TEE formula.

That meant the amount of stored fat her body needed to burn decreased as her weight decreased.

According to the TEE formula, she was taking in – and using – 3345 calories daily at the start of her diet. Reducing her intake by 500 calories, to 2845 calories daily, should result in losing a pound in seven days. And at the beginning, that was what was happening.

But things were different after she lost five pounds. Now she weighed 167, so according to the TEE formula she was burning 3269 calories per day, not 3345. She was still consuming 2845 calories daily, so now she needed to burn 424 calories worth of her stored fat per day, rather than 500. That was equivalent to burning 2954 calories worth of stored fat per week, instead of 3500. She was now losing at a rate of 0.84 pounds per week instead of a pound per week – 13.5 ounces, not sixteen.

After she had lost ten pounds, the problem got worse. Now she was using only 3192 calories per day, according to the formula. But she continued to take in 2845 calories daily, so now she only needed to burn 358 calories worth of stored fat per day, and she was only losing at a rate of about eleven ounces per week.

After she lost 15 pounds, it was down to less than nine ounces per week.

As she continued to lose weight, the number of calories her body needed to get by burning stored fat continued to decrease. With each day that passed, her weight became less, so her daily calorie usage decreased. That meant the amount of stored fat she needed to burn decreased along with it. The more she lost, the slower her weight loss became. As a result, it took about three months longer than she originally expected to reach her 150-pound goal.

This kind of process, where something changes by an amount that is related to its current value, leads to what scientists call an exponential decrease. Exponential decrease is like the fabled train that, each hour, goes halfway from where it is to the next station. Every hour, it gets closer; but every hour, it only gets halfway there. The other half always remains to be covered, so it gets closer and closer but never fully reaches the station.

Exponential decreases occur commonly in nature; for example, it describes the decay of a radioactive element, where the number of atoms that decay per second is proportional to the number of atoms that have not yet decayed. Every time an atom decays, there are fewer atoms left that can decay, so each decay reduces the frequency of decays that follow it.

Norma's weight loss works the same way. Every pound she loses reduces the amount of fat she needs to burn daily, which in turn reduces how much weight she loses the next day. Her rate of weight loss depends on her weight, which means that it results in an exponential decrease.

I call this approach "Exponential Weight Loss" because that's how it works – you lose weight *exponentially.* It's based on using the TEE formula in Chapter 5 to describe how your calorie usage depends on your weight, which makes your calorie shortfall depend on your weight, which in turn makes your weight loss depend on your weight. The formula lets me calculate how your weight decreases as time goes by. The details of that calculation are given in

Appendix B; in this chapter, I'll just use the results to show you what happens.

Norma started out by choosing a daily intake of 2845 calories. That meant that her weight would continue to decrease as long as her daily calorie usage remained greater than the 2845 calories she was consuming daily. According to the TEE equation, using 2845 calories per day corresponds to weighing about 139 pounds. So if Norma continued consuming 2845 calories per day, her weight would decrease exponentially toward 139 pounds – what scientists would call her "asymptotic" weight.* She would get closer and closer to it but, like the train in the example above, she wouldn't ever quite get there – although she would eventually get so close, within a fraction of an ounce, that it wouldn't matter. And the more she lost, the less rapidly she would lose; that's why it took her so much longer than 22 weeks to lose 22 pounds. She assumed she would continue to lose a pound each week, but instead she lost weight exponentially, less and less each week.

For exponential decay, the changing rate of decrease is an important characteristic of the process. It is measured by a time scale that is called a "half-life." A half-life is the amount of time required for the quantity that is decreasing to decrease by one-half of its current value – which is an hour in the story of the train that never reaches the station. After one half-life, it's halfway there. In the second half-life, it goes half of what's left, or a quarter of the initial distance, so it's three-quarters of the way there. After three

---

* When a quantity gets closer and closer to a final value in this fashion, that value is called the *asymptotic value* or *asymptote*.

half-lives, it's seven-eighths. And so on; after eight half-lives, it's less than one-half of one percent of the original distance from the station. It isn't quite there yet; it never will be, but eventually it will get so close that you can hop off and the remaining distance doesn't matter.

The half-life is determined by the quantities involved – in this case, the parameters in the TEE formulas. The half-life for weight loss, based on these formulas, turns out to be about 158 days. That's how long it takes for the decreasing quantity – the difference between Norma's current weight and her asymptotic weight of 139 pounds – to drop by one-half.

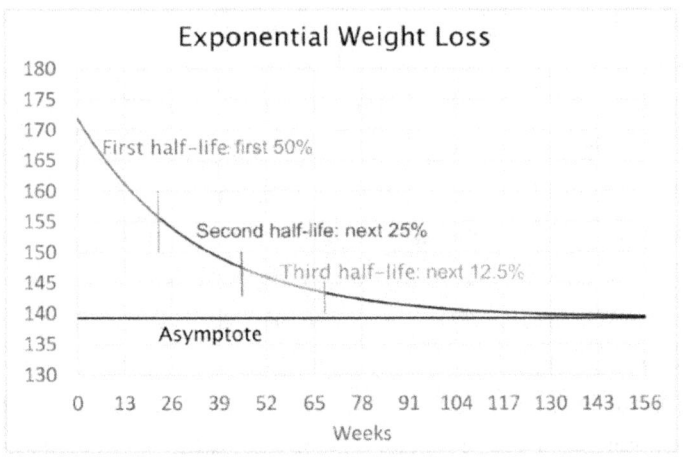

Figure 5. Exponential weight loss toward an asymptote

This exponential weight loss is shown in Figure 5. In the first half-life of 158 days, Norma would lose half of the 33-pound difference between her starting point of 172 pounds and her asymptotic weight of 139 pounds. That means she would lose 16.5 pounds, and at the end of the first half-life, she would weigh 155.5 pounds.

If she continued dieting for another half-life, she would not lose another 15.5 pounds; she would lose half the difference between her new weight, 155.5 pounds, and her asymptotic weight of 139 pounds. So she would lose 8.25 pounds, taking her down to 147.25 pounds.

She reached her 150-pound goal before that happened, but if she had continued, she would lose halfway from 147.25 to 139 during the third half-life. And so on. With each half-life, she would get halfway from where she was when it started to her asymptotic value of 139 pounds. And in each half-life, she would lose only half as much as in the preceding one.

This "law of diminishing returns" is disheartening, and that may be why some dieters lose their zeal long before they lose the amount of weight their diets would eventually lead to. The long half-life of 158 days makes losing weight a very slow process.

Why is the half-life so long? The number is determined by the ratio of the 3500 calories contained in a pound of fat to the 15.3 calories per day required to support one pound of weight. That is a large number, so the half-life is large. If fat contained fewer calories per pound, or our bodies needed more calories per pound, we could lose weight faster. But we can't change either of those numbers, and that makes weight loss slow unless the calorie reduction is huge, as in the plans described in Chapter 4.

What basic metabolic science tells us, then, is that your weight changes exponentially, with a long half-life, when your calorie balance changes. When Norma removed 500 calories from her daily calorie intake, her body responded by beginning an exponential decrease toward the weight level that her new calorie intake would support.

That's what had happened to me years back when I began running. Rather than reducing my calorie intake, I increased my calorie usage. That shifted my body's balance toward using more calories than my intake would support, so I lost weight. Exercise science has studied the extra energy required for running and found that it also is proportional to your weight, which meant that my weight loss from running was also exponential. The same is true for other forms of exercise, as described in Appendix C.

But regardless of how it happens, an imbalance between the calories you use and the calories you take in will cause your weight to change exponentially toward the level corresponding to the calories you take in. You won't lose at a fixed rate of pounds per week; instead, your rate of loss will decrease as your weight decreases. That will make it take much longer to reach your goal than you might expect.

Ultimately, however, your final weight will be determined by your final calorie intake, via the TEE formula. If you want your weight to be stable at a new level, your calorie intake must be stable at a level corresponding to it. You can't diet for a while and then go back to your previous eating habits; if you do, you'll just start gaining exponentially until you reach your previous weight.

What nutritional research has shown, then, is that weight loss is an exponential change with a long half-life. If your calorie usage exceeds your calorie intake for any reason, your body will begin to restore the balance by

using its stored fat. That will result in an exponential weight loss with an asymptote corresponding to about one pound for each 15.3 calories, but the rate of change will correspond to a long half-life of 158 days. Unfortunately, however, the same thing happens in reverse if your calorie intake exceeds your calorie usage; you will gain weight exponentially. In the next chapter I'll show you how that happens.

Chapter 7
The Yo-Yo Diet Plan

Americans have been dieting for years, losing pound after pound, and then regaining it, as described in Chapter 4. In this chapter, I want to show you how that happens in more detail, based on understanding weight change as an exponential process.

Unfortunately, dieting has come to mean a short-term change in what you eat. You diet for a while, and then it's over and you can go back to eating as you used to. You don't need to diet forever; once it's finished, life can return to "normal."

Most people, having reached the target weight they set (or, perhaps, a weight they decide is low enough, even if it isn't the target) will go back to eating as they did before the diet. They may even eat a bit more, to make up for having gone hungry for so long. They have deprived themselves of some things they enjoy for quite a while, weeks or months, and they think they deserve to relax and recover. After all, who wants to keep on eating those monotonous diet meals if you no longer need to?

And when they do, they start regaining the weight they lost, for all the physiological and psychological reasons described in Chapter 4. But regaining the weight is an exponential process, just as losing it was. If your calorie intake exceeds your calorie usage, you will gain weight exponentially, with the same 158-day half-life as when you lose weight.

Let's assume that's what Norma did. After losing 22 pounds, she congratulated herself for successfully dieting, even though it took much longer than expected. But now she could stop dieting and live normally again. So she went back to her earlier lifestyle, consuming her earlier intake of 3345 calories per day.

And when she did, she started gaining back the weight she had lost. Her new 150-pound body requires only 3009 calories per day, according to the TEE formula. It doesn't need 3345 calories. So she is now taking in 336 calories more than she is using. That means she will start storing 336 calories of excess intake daily as fat.

Now, 336 calories per day isn't a lot, compared to the thousands of calories of reduction required by the diet plans in Chapter 4. At 3500 calories per pound of fat, it means gaining just an ounce and a half of fat daily. But as her body starts storing that extra fat, her weight starts climbing back toward where it started. As time goes by, that gain accumulates in the same exponential way that her lost weight disappeared during the diet.

Her weight will change as shown in Figure 6. After having lost twenty-two pounds in thirty-seven weeks, she will gain back about ten pounds of the twenty-two she lost within the next four and a half months. As time goes by, she gets closer and closer to the asymptotic weight that corresponds to the 3345 calories per day she's consuming – which is 172 pounds, right back where she started out.

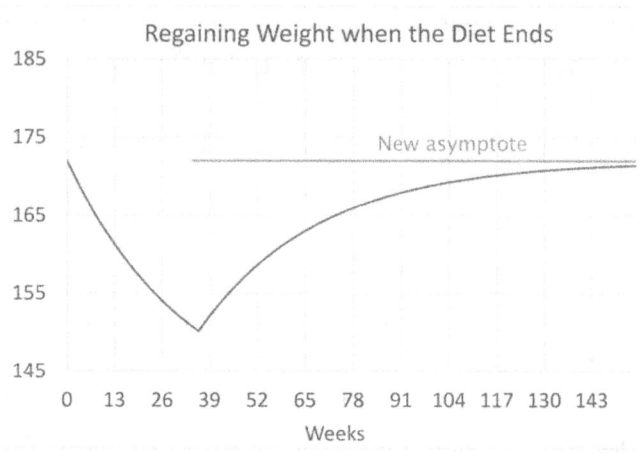

Figure 6. Norma goes back to "normal" eating and gains toward a new asymptote

It's the mirror image of losing weight – her weight increases toward 172 pounds, the weight her original 3345-calorie intake supported. She's now gaining exponentially the extra weight her earlier calorie intake supported. It's exponential weight gain rather than exponential weight loss. In the first half-life of 158 days after she stops dieting, she gains back half of the 22 pounds she lost. She gains another quarter of that much in the next half-life. As time goes by, her weight goes back up, getting closer and closer to where she started.

In less than five months after getting down to 150 pounds, Norma is back up to 160 pounds. Having regained almost half of what she lost, she knows what she needs to do – get back on a diet. This time she goes on Nutrisystem, and in five weeks she is back down to 150 pounds. Nutrisystem worked, she thinks to herself.

And it did, for five weeks; but then she pronounces herself successful again and stops dieting. She goes back to eating like a 172-pounder, and her weight starts climbing again toward that level. After another five months, she is back up to 160 pounds, so it's back to Nutrisystem. As before, she loses ten pounds in five weeks; but then she stops dieting, and starts gaining it back again. She can't maintain 150 pounds on a 172-pound menu, so the process has to be repeated again and again.

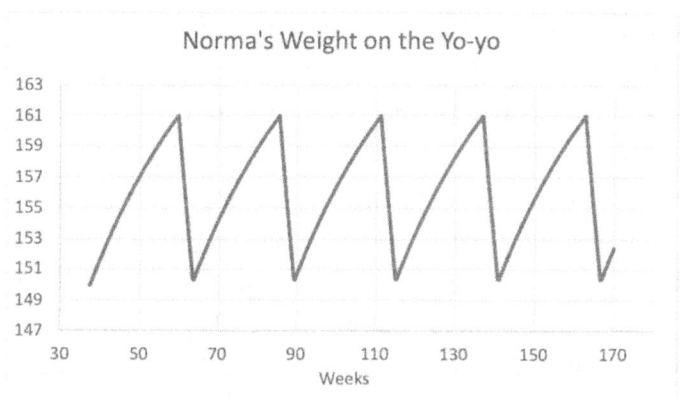

Figure 7. The yo-yo cycle

And so she continues on the cycle, losing weight for five weeks and then gaining it back during the next five months, over and over, as shown in Figure 7. She becomes a regular

Nutrisystem customer, valued by them as proof that their plan works.

She has become addicted to dieting.

It's a common occurrence. Researchers at Columbia University found that 73% of their study subjects reported losing and regaining a minimum of 10 pounds at least once – and some cycled the weight up to 20 times in their lifetime. According to data reported in a study by the University of Colorado, 35% of people who start by dieting occasionally become addicted to dieting.

This pattern is often called "yo-yo dieting" and it is seriously unhealthy. It's linked to heart disease, insulin resistance, higher blood pressure, inflammation, diabetes, fatty liver, and gallstones. All the health problems described earlier as associated with rapid weight loss are exacerbated by yo-yo dieting.

In addition to these negative effects on your health, yo-yo dieting can have a serious impact on your self-esteem. Every time you regain weight, you may feel like you're a failure. According to studies, yo-yo dieting can lead to feelings of ineffectiveness as well as negative psychological and behavioral consequences such as depression, anger, anxiety, and feelings of guilt. Repeating the yo-yo cycle can make you believe that you are a failure who lacks the strength to keep the weight off. It can also affect your relationship with others, and in turn, make you feel isolated and unworthy.

Dieting is not a pleasant process, and few of us have the patience to stick to a diet for very long. So diet plans like the ones analyzed in Chapter 4 are structured to make you lose weight quickly, by creating a large reduction in your caloric intake. They want you to tell other people how successful you were, and how much you lost, so they will buy into the plan too.

But they know that you will re-gain the weight after you stop dieting and need to buy their product again. That's how they make money. Yo-yo dieters like Norma are their favorite customers.

The real problem with the commercial diets, then, is that you can't stay on them – eventually you have to stop. If you don't, you'll keep losing weight until you become seriously malnourished. But when you stop, you regain the weight.

How can you lose weight but avoid the yo-yo?

There are two ways. One is not to "return to normal" when the diet ends, but to adopt a "new normal" that corresponds to your new weight. Instead of going back to 3345 calories daily, Norma would adopt a new eating plan with only 3009 calories, the amount her slimmer 150-pound body uses daily.

The other is simply to start off at that reduced calorie level in the first place and let your body adapt to it. Instead of dieting strenuously at first and mildly later, you begin with a much smaller calorie reduction corresponding to the weight target you choose and simply maintain it.

How much smaller? As I've shown in Chapter 6, your body only needs about 15.3 calories for each pound you weigh. To lose 22 pounds, as Norma wanted to do, you only need to cut 337 calories out of your daily intake. That's a tiny amount compared to the thousands of calories required by the commercial diet plans. You won't lose the weight as quickly as you might have on Nutrisystem or Weight Watchers, but you won't have to suffer through their painful food deprivation or risk damage to your health. Instead, you'll set a new calorie intake level at the beginning, and all you have to do is just maintain it.

And if you do that, you don't have to worry about what to do later, because there is no later; you've adopted a new eating plan for good. That is the beauty of exponential weight loss. Instead of a temporary but extreme diet, you make a small but permanent change in your eating habits.

Either way, you can avoid the yo-yo only by reducing your calorie intake permanently so that it corresponds to your target weight. That's the simple truth about weight loss – it's only permanent if the calorie reduction is permanent. It doesn't matter whether you make that reduction in two weeks or two years. What does matter is that you can't go back to eating as you did before the diet, or you will gain back the weight you lost.

So what do the commercial diet plans accomplish? Quick temporary weight loss for you, huge profits for the diet business. In the long term, you wind up back where you started, or worse. If you want to *weigh less in the long term*, rather than just lose weight temporarily, you must find a way to reduce your calorie intake permanently. You can't just lose weight for a while and then go back to eating as you did before – if you do, the lost weight will return. That's what has happened to all those people who spent all that money on diets that ultimately didn't produce the result they were after.

Now you can understand why diets don't work, and why more than $72,000,000,000 spent every year on diets is wasted. The diets lead to losing weight while you're on them, but the weight comes back when you stop. Rather than creating a leaner, healthier population, they have created a nation of yo-yo dieting addicts.

If *weighing less* is the objective, rather than simply losing weight, then none of those plans work. To lose weight and keep it off requires long-term calorie reduction; you can't lose long-term weight on a short-term diet. But the size of the calorie reduction is tiny, compared to what the commercial diets require. That makes the process both easy and healthy. In Chapter 8, I'll tell you how that worked for me, so that you can do it too.

Chapter 8
How to Weigh Less

Now that you understand how exponential weight loss works, I want to share with you my own successful weight-loss experience.

For me, successfully weighing less began with the visit to the doctor that I mentioned at the beginning of this book. He told me two things. The first was that I needed to lose some weight. The second was that, based on his general health questionnaire, I was drinking more alcohol than I should.

My wife and I usually had two or three glasses of wine in the late afternoon, just before dinner or with it. I certainly didn't think of that as "too much alcohol," although I knew I should not drink it if I expected to drive later. We weren't drinking because we were thirsty or because we craved it; it was just a pleasant way to end the day and begin the evening. It was a habit. A pleasant one, but still just a habit. And although I was confident that I was neither "Obese" nor alcoholic, having the two issues juxtaposed made me realize that they had a single simple solution.

I realized that I could solve both those problems if I would give up that wine habit. Giving it up, even forever, wasn't that profound a change in my daily life, and I certainly wouldn't be thirsty without it. Even so, I wanted to be certain that the result would be worth the change. So I did the calculation that follows.

A five-ounce glass of wine contains about 123 calories. By eliminating two glasses of wine, I would reduce my daily caloric intake by 246 calories, without reducing my daily activity level. As a result, I would lose weight, just as if I had gone on a "two-fewer-glasses-of-wine" diet.

The question was, how much weight would I lose by giving up two glasses of wine? Compared to the thousands of calories required by Nutrisystem or Weight Watchers, a reduction of 246 calories hardly seemed like enough to do much good.

To find out, I went to the TEE formulas. If you turn them inside out, they tell you precisely how your weight depends on your daily calorie intake:

Weight in pounds =
> **Calories consumed per day/15.3**
> $-$ (46.7 for women, 63.9 for men)

Look at that formula closely. The first term is in bold because it's the one that matters; it relates my weight to my daily calorie consumption. If I decrease the number of calories I consume per day by 15.3, that term becomes smaller by one pound. My daily calorie intake won't be enough to support one pound of my weight, so I'll need to burn stored fat to make up for it. That means my weight will decrease by one pound as well!

I only needed to reduce my daily intake by about 15.3 calories for each pound I want to lose, according to the TEE formulas. That's tiny, compared to my total calorie intake. It's the number of calories in *five-eighths of an ounce* of wine. Not a glass. Barely more than a spoonful! At 15.3 calories per pound, two glasses of wine were responsible for *sixteen pounds* of fat on my body.

Could this be true? Could I really lose sixteen pounds, just by giving up two glasses of wine?

As surprising as it seems, that is the inevitable result of the science behind the TEE formulas. Extending the Mifflin-St Jeor group's REE measurements as described in Chapter 5 leads directly to the conclusion that the average American requires about 15.3 calories of energy to support each pound of weight. If you reduce your caloric intake by 15.3 calories, your body will not be getting enough energy to support your current weight, so you will burn a pound of stored fat to get your calorie usage back in balance with your calorie intake.

I would lose about one pound for every 15.3 calories by which I reduced your daily intake. Just 15.3 calories per pound per day. That's all it takes. I had never realized that it took such a small change to lose a pound.

By giving up two glasses of wine – 246 calories – I could expect to lose somewhere in the vicinity of sixteen pounds.

Could I do without that wine? Of course I could, especially since I wanted to reduce my alcohol consumption anyway. It was part of a pleasant interlude in my late afternoon, but not something I really needed. I could easily switch to water or diet soda. My wife didn't object – she continued having some wine, although perhaps a bit less than before, and she wasn't concerned about the weight loss involved. So we still celebrate the end of the day, but I do it without the alcohol – and its calories.

I gave up my daily wine and my weight started dropping. I didn't need to go on Weight Watchers or Nutrisystem and cut my daily calories by thousands. All I needed to do was eliminate two or three glasses of wine from my daily diet to see a significant weight loss.

In two years I lost over twenty pounds, as shown in Figure 8.[*] Analyzing my progress as an exponential decrease suggests that my weight loss corresponds to an asymptote of about twenty-one pounds lost, based on a calorie reduction of about 320 calories per day, about 2½ glasses of wine worth. My actual weight loss corresponded to one pound for every 15.1 calories, a bit better than I expected.

---

[*] There were times, of course, when I didn't avoid wine, or even follow my normal diet – holidays, or going on a two-week cruise with lots of food and wine included. I omitted these days, and the following days recovering from them, from my calculations.

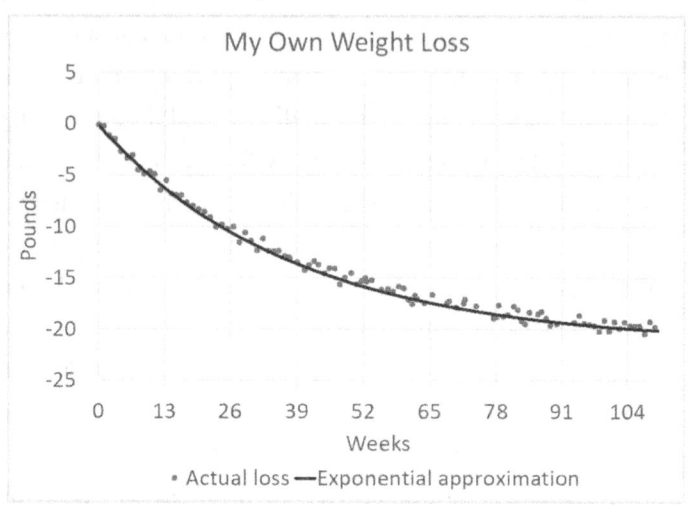

Figure 8. My weight loss after giving up my daily wine

It wasn't quick, as it would have been if I had cut my daily calorie intake by thousands on Weight Watchers or Nutrisystem; it was slow, starting out at an imperceptible two-thirds of an ounce per day. It took over two weeks to lose the first pound. The day-to-day fluctuations in my weight made that first pound hard to see, but I could tell that overall I was a pound or so lighter. And as time went by, I got closer and closer to my asymptotic weight. It took about two years for me to lose 95% of the predicted amount; since then, my weight has stayed near that asymptote, varying day-to-day as described in Chapter 2.

At that point, I considered myself a success. I knew that exponential weight loss would not bring me all the way to my asymptotic weight, just closer and closer to it. Losing the last 5% wasn't all that important. I knew that my weight would hover around its new level and gradually drop those last few ounces.

This was not a diet; it was a change in my eating and drinking habits. I no longer expect to drink two glasses of wine before dinner. I no longer have that habit. I have no expectation of "returning to normal" – this *is* my normal now.

You can do this too.

The first step is to decide how much weight you want to lose. You may want to aim for a slightly larger figure since the weight loss is exponential – you won't ever lose the full amount, but you'll get very close to it in two years. Then estimate how many calories you need to cut from your daily intake based on about one pound for every 15.3 calories.

It doesn't need to be starvation – just 150 calories, the amount in a can of soda, will result in losing about ten pounds in two years. You don't have to change your eating pattern drastically and cut out thousands of calories the way Weight Watchers or Nutrisystem would require. A small change in your overall eating and drinking habits will let you weigh whatever amount you choose within about two years. It doesn't have to be your late-afternoon wine, as it was for me; choose whatever you will miss least and eliminate its calories.

Table II shows some examples of things that you might give up, along with their calories and the approximate amount of weight you would lose if you removed them from your daily eating habit. The amounts given are the exponential weight loss you should expect in two years, based on losing one pound for every 15.3 calories:

Give up:	Serving size	Calories	Two-year weight loss
Soda	12-ounce can	157	9.8
Whiskey	1.5 fluid ounces	105	6.8
Beer	12-ounce can	145	9.0
Wine	1 5-ounce glass	123	7.6
Potato chips	1-ounce serving	155	9.6
Sugar	1 teaspoon	16	1.0
Coffee cream	1 tbsp. heavy cream	52	3.2
Toast with butter and jam	1 slice	125	7.8
French Fries	4-ounce serving	365	22.7
Burrito	medium with beef, beans & cheese	628	39.0
Premium hamburger	7.6-ounce two-patty sandwich	563	34.9
Chocolate cookies	3 standard cookies	159	9.9
Donut	1 glazed donut	269	16.7
Ice cream	1 cup	274	17.0
Caffe Latte	16 ounces	190	11.8
Candy bar	1 ounce	148	9.2

Table II. Exponential weight loss for various calorie reductions

You can choose one of these, or combine several of them, or choose something else – just look up the number of calories it contains. All that matters is that the calories add up to approximately 15.3 times the amount of weight you want to lose.

Some people habitually start the day with a full breakfast; skipping one slice of buttered toast with jam will lead to a two-year loss of nearly eight pounds, and it's not likely that you will be noticeably hungrier before lunch. (Eat the buttered toast but skip the jam and you'll lose close to two pounds.)

Stop using cream in your coffee and lose about three pounds; switch to half-and-half (20 calories) and lose about two pounds.

If you have a soda every day at lunch, switch to diet soda and lose nine pounds. Or if you munch on potato chips while you watch television, skip them and lose the same amount.

If you usually have a bowl of ice cream at the end of the evening, going without it won't leave you hungry but it will let you lose over sixteen pounds.

In two years, exponential weight loss will result in your dropping about ten pounds for every 150 calories you stop taking in. It may be a bit more or a bit less than ten pounds, depending on your metabolism; but it will be close to that much.

The way to weigh less, then, is simply this: eliminate a few hundred calories from your daily eating habits. Give up something you can easily do without, or replace it with something that has fewer calories. It can be a glass of wine, or a slice of toast. Switch a can of soda to water or diet soda. Leave out dessert after lunch. Quit nibbling on potato chips, or replace them with something with fewer calories.

Just about fifteen calories for each pound you want to lose. A small reduction in calories produces a big reduction in weight.

The approach I've just described is significantly different from the commercial diet plans in two ways. First of all, it relies on a much smaller, easier change in what you eat. But more importantly, it requires you to make that change permanently. That is the hard part. The truth is that you are not just eating less; you are making a fundamental change in your eating habits. It's a small change, compared to what the commercial diets require; but it's a change. And changing habits is not easy.

You need perseverance and patience. Perseverance, since you need to follow this new regimen forever; patience, because it doesn't happen quickly. It happens exponentially, with a half-life of 158 days.

If you reduce your daily calorie intake by the 246 calories contained in two glasses of wine, as I did, you will ultimately lose about sixteen pounds, although you will initially lose only less than an ounce per day. You won't even notice that, especially since your weight is fluctuating daily by several pounds anyway. In twenty-four days, you will have lost about 10% of your target amount. In five months, after about one half-life, you will have lost half of the weight you will eventually lose.

That will be rewarding; but you'll now be losing at only half the rate you started with. The fact that your weight loss slows as you go can be disappointing, but keep in mind that in two years you will weigh about sixteen pounds less. And since this is a forever weight loss plan, taking that long is not a problem.

You could lose weight more quickly with a commercial diet plan. But when you reach your target weight, you would still have to reduce your long-term calorie intake by that same amount, 246 calories, if you want to maintain that weight rather than regain it. Either way, you have to remove 246 calories permanently from your daily eating habit, or you will gain back the weight you lost. To me, it was much easier just to make that change to start with, and not suffer through the extreme-low-calorie diet.

What's essential, if you want to use a commercial quick-weight-loss plan, to start by identifying what you are going to eliminate permanently from your daily eating habits. Any diet plan that says it has an ending point – such as "Lose thirteen pounds in four weeks" – can't lead to permanent weight loss, because it ends. When the "four weeks" is up, and the diet is over, you will regain the weight you lost unless you reduce your calorie intake to match your new weight.

You must decide at the beginning that you are making a permanent change in your eating habits. If you don't, it's almost a certainty that afterwards you will go back to eating as you did before. And when you eat what you ate before, you will eventually weigh what you weighed before. To keep from regaining weight, start the diet by identifying about 15 calories per pound from you are permanently eliminating from your daily eating pattern. Then, whether you lose weight exponentially or more quickly, you will achieve your long-term weight goal.

You can't lose long-term weight with a short-term plan. Commercial diet plans with big calorie reductions bring about quick, but temporary, weight loss. They won't lead to weighing less in the long term. A small reduction in daily calories is all that's required to weigh significantly less permanently. You don't have to suffer by cutting out 2000 calories a day; you can choose your target weight loss, and then cut out about fifteen calories per pound. But what weight should you choose? In the next chapter, I'll tell you how to make that decision.

Chapter 9
How Much Should You Weigh?

The first step in the process of successfully weighing less, of course, is to decide how much you want to weigh. Not how much you *need* to weigh, according to the CDC or your doctor or the diet industry. How much do you *want* to weigh? In this chapter I'll suggest a basis for your choice.

Wanting to do something is not the same as needing to do something. Wanting comes from inside you; needing is externally imposed. When you do something because you *need* to do it, it creates stress. To avoid unpleasant stress, you are likely to respond by not doing it. When you do something because you *want* to do it, there is less stress because the choice was yours.

My doctor told me that I was "Obese" by the standards dictated by the CDC. The CDC said I needed to get to their "Normal or Healthy Level" by reducing my BMI to 25[*]. To

---

[*] The BMI is actually a spurious measure; weight should be proportional to volume – the cube of the height, not the square.

reach that level I would need to lose over 50 pounds – about a quarter of my body weight. That would be a huge undertaking, but the CDC said that I needed to lose it or I would be facing serious health problems.

Losing weight was not necessarily something I *wanted* to do; it was something the doctor, and the CDC, told me I *needed* to do. Their intent, of course, was for me to weigh less in order to avoid risking serious health problems. But I was dubious about whether I was really "Obese," and my previous experience with diets made me doubt that dieting would work. So I could not make the intellectual leap necessary to convert what the doctor said I *needed* to do into something I *wanted* to do. Instead, I decided to explore the relationship between the CDC's ratings and reality.

Is the average person unhealthy because of obesity? The CDC certainly thinks so. By their reckoning, in 2017–18,

- 9.2% of Americans were "Severely or Morbidly Obese" (BMI greater than 40)
- 33.2% of Americans were "Obese" (BMI between 30 and 40)
- 28.9% of Americans were "Overweight" (BMI between 25 and 30)
- 27.2% of Americans were "Normal or Healthy" (BMI between 18.5 and 25)

By using the square, the BMI overestimates an accurate measure for those above average height and underestimates it for those below average. But the CDC has made the BMI the definitive guide for determining if someone is overweight, and after fifty years it's too late to change it.

- 1.5% were "Underweight" (BMI less than 18.5) as shown in Figure 9.

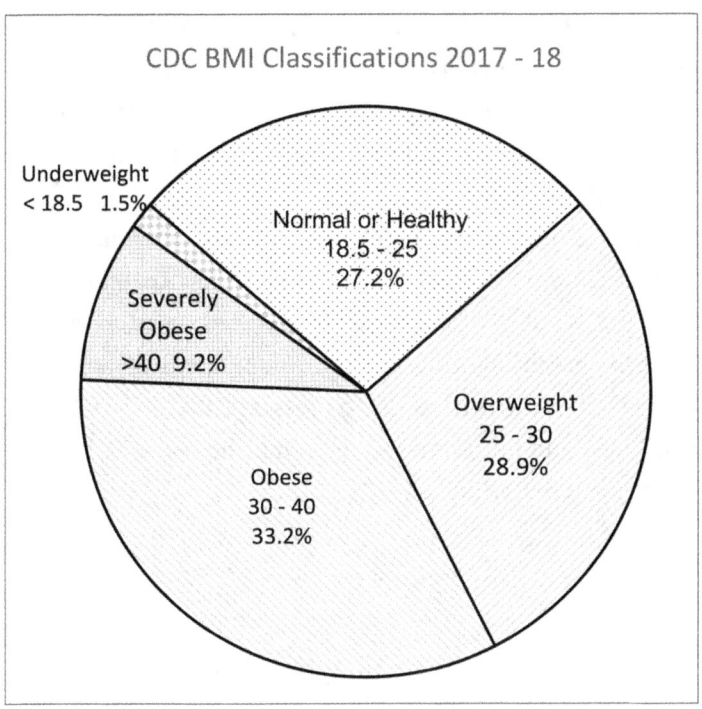

Figure 9. The CDC's classifications of health status based on the BMI (data from www.cdc.gov/nchs/data/databriefs/db360-h.pdf)

Their definitions implied that 71.3% of Americans – almost three out of four – were too heavy to be considered "Normal or Healthy." This portion has increased steadily, from 44.8% in 1962 to 71.3% in 2017–18. The percentage who are "Obese" or "Severely Obese" increased from 13.3% to 42.4% during the same period.

Based on the average weights given earlier and average heights measured by the CDC, the average American has a BMI of 29.4; women currently have a BMI of 29.7 and men a BMI of 29.2. Both men and women are at the top of the "Overweight" category and very nearly "Obese." To reach the "Normal or Healthy" level of 25 would require the average American man to lose 31 pounds and the average American woman to lose 28 pounds.

If all of this is true, barely one-fourth of the individuals in the USA are "Normal or Healthy." It's hard to understand how the word "Normal" can be applied to a group that includes barely one-fourth of the population. If anything, the ones with a BMI of 25 or less are the ones who are abnormal, and the normal American is the one who is in the overweight majority.

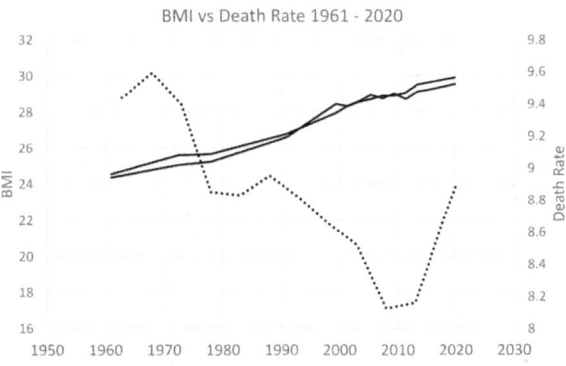

Figure 10. Death rates versus average BMIs (BMIs from www.cdc.gov/nchs/data/nhsr/nhsr122-508.pdf; death rates from www.macrotrends.net/countries/USA/united-states/death-rate)

It's even harder to understand how more than one-fourth of the population can have become seriously unhealthy because of excess weight during the last fifty years. You would think that an increase in the number of unhealthy people from 44.8% in 1962 to 71.3% in 2017–18 would be reflected in a parallel increase in the number of deaths. Yet, as shown in Figure 10, the overall death rate actually decreased by about 15% during that same time period. That is hardly consistent with the CDC's statement that "Obesity is epidemic in the United States today and a major cause of death."

The principal claim made to support the idea that increased weight brings decreased health and earlier death is that obesity is associated with a number of "comorbidities" – that is, that death rates from various diseases increase with increasing weight. With these diseases, they say, the more you weigh, the sooner you die. But even if the health problems associated with some diseases increase as weight increases, the increase does not become suddenly worse at a BMI of 30; it increases only gradually, not abruptly. Rather than creating panic by suggesting that people are at grave risk if they have BMI's in the range questionably called "Obese", it would be more accurate to say simply that the risk of these health problems increases gradually with the BMI. A correlation isn't the same as an epidemic.

In fact, however, the available research shows no sign of epidemic growth in obesity but instead reveal a small gradual shift in which many people moved from BMI's just below 25 to BMI's in the lower part of the 25–30 range, along with a similar small shift from just below 30 into the low 30s. That's a small shift, not an epidemic, by any reasonable definition of epidemic growth.

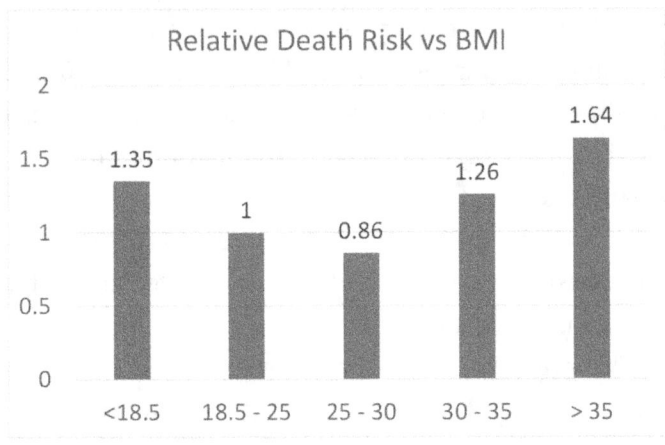

Figure 11. Relative death risk versus BMI (data from National Center for Health Statistics, Series 3, #42)

And the relationship between death rates and the BMI does not show that the "Normal or Healthy" group are in fact the healthiest Americans. The CDC's own National Center for Health Statistics evaluated the relative risk of death as a function of BMI, with the results shown in Figure 11. Those labeled "Overweight" by the CDC, with BMI values between 25 and 30, have a death risk that is only 86% of that of those the CDC deems "Healthy or Normal."

If being healthy means having less risk of dying, then the CDC's own results show that the group it calls "Overweight" are 14% healthier than those it calls "Normal or Healthy"! To me, that suggests that the CDC's definition of a "Normal or Healthy" BMI is not realistic and needs to be revised. A new categorization of health versus BMI should be adopted that more accurately corresponds to the relative death risk associated with the BMI.

In my opinion, the healthiest people are those with the lowest risk of death. I would call you healthy if you are less likely to die than the average person. In other words, I suggest that "Healthy" should be used to describe people whose risk of death relative to their weight is in the lower half of the entire population.

The least healthy people are those whose death risk in in the top 10% of the population. This group includes both the excessively heavy, whom I would call "Dangerously Overweight" rather than morbidly obese, and the excessively thin who are "Dangerously Underweight."

The remaining 40% consists of those whose death risk is greater than 50% of the population but less than the highest 10%. They should be considered simply "Overweight" or "Underweight."

These ranges can be estimated by combining the data shown in Figure 11 with the distribution of the population as a function of BMI shown in Figure 9. The result of this calculation, the percentile ranking of death risk corresponding to different values of the BMI, is shown in Figure 12.

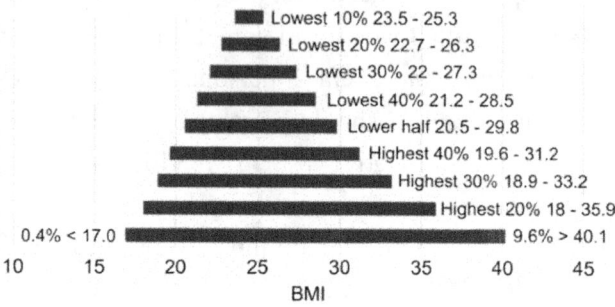

Figure 12. The BMI ranges corresponding to death risk percentile ranges, based on the CDC data

This result shows the BMI ranges that correspond to various percentile rankings for death risk. For example, the 10% of the population with the lowest death risk, represented by the top bar, are those with BMI's between 23.5 and 25.2. The healthiest half of the population consists of those whose death risk percentile ranking is less than 50%; that is, they are less likely to die, based on their weight, than 50% of the total population. I would call this group "Healthy."[*] It includes those with BMI's between 20.7 and 29.8.

The least healthy are those whose death risk is greatest – those who have a death risk that puts them in the percentile range above 90%. These are the 10% not

---

[*] Not "Normal and Healthy" – an individual of "normal weight" would weigh the average amount, which might be very different from one that is healthy.

included in the "< 90%" range in the figure – those with BMI's greater than 40.1 (9.6%) or less than 17.0 (0.4%). They face the most significant risk of death associated with their weight. I would call these groups "Dangerously Overweight" and "Dangerously Underweight."

The remaining 40% are those with BMI's between 29.8 and 40.1 (33.7%) or between 17.0 and 20.7 (6.3%), whom I would call "Overweight," and "Underweight" respectively.

These percentile ranges provide a far more realistic assessment of the nation's health than the CDC's current categories and should replace them:

- "Dangerously Overweight" (BMI greater than 40.1): 9.6% of Americans
- "Overweight" (BMI between 29.8 and 40.1): 33.7% of Americans
- "Healthy" (BMI between 20.7 and 29.8): 50% of Americans
- "Underweight" (BMI between 17.0 and 20.7): 6.3% of Americans
- "Dangerously Underweight" (BMI less than 17.0): 0.4% of Americans

These categories and their associated BMI ranges are shown in Figure 13.

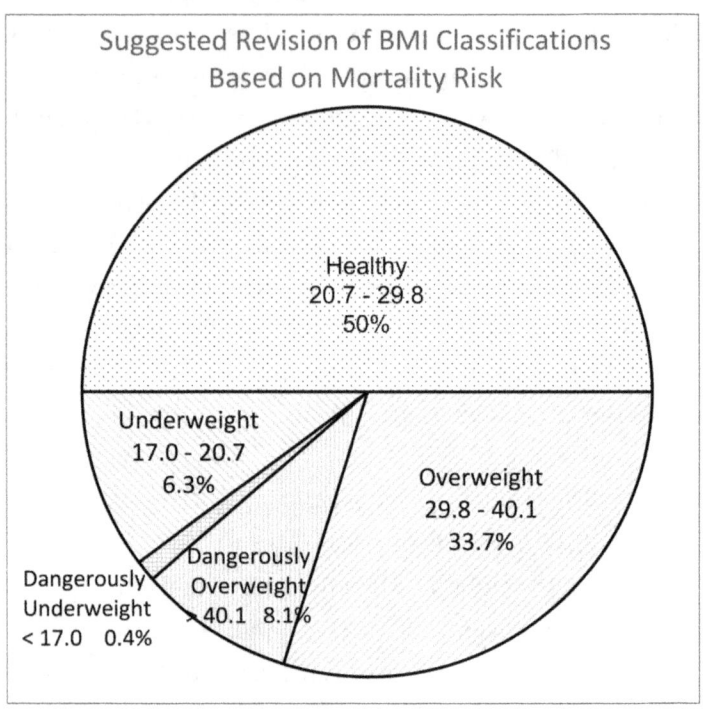

Figure 13. BMI Categories based on death risk

The "Healthy" group includes the average American, whose BMI of 29.4 is healthier than 54% of the American population. Rather than being "Overweight" and nearly "Obese," as the current classification scheme would indicate, the average person is in the healthier half of the population.

The average American woman, with a BMI of 29.7, is not borderline "Obese"; she is in the 47th percentile of risk – that is, 53% of the population has a higher death risk than she does. She is in the healthier half of the population if she weighs between 130 and 180. A healthy daily intake for her is between 2700 and 3460 calories, rather than 1600 to 2400 as the CDC recommends.

The average American man, with a BMI of 29.2, is even better off, with a death risk lower than that of about 55% of the overall population. He is in the healthier half of the population if he weighs between 155 and 210. A healthy daily intake for him is between 3300 and 4200 calories, rather than 2000 to 3000 as the CDC recommends.

The "Dangerously Overweight" group with BMI's above 40.1 roughly corresponds to the 9.2% of Americans with a BMI greater than 40 who were in the CDC category called "Severely Obese" in 2017-18. It would include men of average height weighing more than 275 pounds and women of average height weighing more than 235 pounds. Their relative death risk is more than 289% of the national average.

It is this group about whom the CDC should be raising concern – those whose weight suggests a significant risk of dying. It hardly seems accurate to say that an average American, who has a BMI of 29.4 and a below-average risk of dying, is facing a "grave" health threat. It would seem more realistic to say that the degree of risk becomes a health crisis only when it's far above average.

But the CDC and other health agencies continue to use their faulty measure and proclaim that there is an obesity crisis. As a result, most primary-care doctors calculate the BMI for every patient who visits them and tell them that they are "Overweight" if it exceeds 25 and "Obese" if it is over 30, suggesting that they are seriously at risk because of their weight. And thanks to the negative connotations of the word "Obese," those same people have developed a negative self-image that makes them think their worth as individuals depends on getting rid of their supposedly excess weight. As a result, a large number of Americans, persuaded that their health and well-being depend on losing weight, have become compulsive dieters.

The time has come for a new understanding of weight – of what it means to be healthy and what it means to be happy with your body. A BMI of 30 does not mean that you are obese or abnormal or unhealthy or unappealing. It doesn't mean that you are going to die soon of one of those diseases that supposedly are epidemic among those with BMI's above 25. It doesn't mean that you need to start buying prepackaged low-calorie meals or running five miles a day. All that it means is that you are about as heavy, for your height, as most Americans, and consequently that you are about as healthy, and as worthwhile, as most Americans.

The CDC needs to adopt a new, realistic categorization of health versus BMI. The pejorative label "Obese" should be scrapped. More accurate descriptions should be based upon the actual health of individuals, as reflected in their relative mortality risk.

With this redefinition, the BMI would provide a much more realistic assessment of the nation's health, based upon the mortality risk associated with increased weight. Rather than reinforcing the diet industry's profit base, the CDC would help the public understand the extent to which their health actually depends on their weight. That kind of understanding would allow my doctor to make a credible recommendation when he says I *need* to lose weight, and for me to decide whether I *want* to lose weight.

Regardless of what the CDC says, I am *not* obese. My BMI is now 29.4, which puts my mortality risk from weight in the healthier half of the population. I don't need to lose 50 pounds to reach the CDC's artificial "Normal or Healthy" – in fact, my death risk would increase if I did!

What I *want* is to weigh somewhere in the middle of the range that has a lower than average death risk. In other words, I want my weight to correspond to a BMI less than 29.8.

Contrary to the CDC's recommendations, you do not need to be extremely thin, with a BMI below 25, to be healthy; if fact, you would be less healthy than the average American. The healthiest people are the 50% of the population who have BMI's between 20.7 and 29.8; they have less mortality risk than the other half of the population. The weight you want to achieve and maintain is one which puts you in this healthier half of the population. You can reach this weight easily and healthily via exponential weight loss. In the next – and final – chapter, I'm going to share some insights I've acquired into making that as easy as possible.

Chapter 10
Weight Loss that Lasts

The science presented in this book has shown that you can achieve a healthy weight exponentially by making a surprisingly small reduction in your daily calorie intake. But that reduction must be a long-term change in your eating habits, rather than a short-term commercial diet. Changing a habit can be painful, even if it's a small change. So in this chapter I want to share some information aimed at helping you succeed in making your weight loss last.

The important first step in achieving a healthy weight is to decide how much you *want* to weigh – not how much the CDC and the diet companies say you *need* to weigh. How much you *want* to weigh depends on two things. One is rational, based on what weight makes you healthiest. The other is emotional, based on your self-image.

Choosing rationally means aiming for the lowest mortality risk. According to the results shown in Chapter 9, that means you want a BMI between 20.7 and 29.8. You will be healthier than average if you weigh somewhere in that range. If your BMI is above 29.8, as mine was, weighing less will allow you to live a healthier life – which in turn contributes to a happier life. You are doing it for yourself, for rational reasons.

The second reason, more emotionally driven, is choosing how much you want to weigh because of how you see yourself and how you think others see you. That is important to many people. But it's also important to remember that you are not just an image; you are the substance of who you are. Your self-image should be based on thinking of yourself as someone who can do what is in your best interest, rather than simply in how you think others might describe you.

Whether your reasons are rational, emotional, or both, you can choose how much you want to weigh, and you can achieve that weight by following the exponential weight loss plan described in Chapter 8. The question is, how do you make that actually happen? It's easy to talk about giving up a glass of wine that you've been enjoying every day at five o'clock. Actually doing it is something else entirely – it's changing a habit that is an enjoyable part of life.

Most of us in the modern world, thankfully, don't eat because our bodies are seriously low on fuel. We fill the car's gas tank only when it gets down close to empty, but we fill our fat tanks several times a day – at every meal and snack. Maybe your standard breakfast is an egg, two slices of bacon, orange juice, and buttered toast. Or you always have a soda with lunch. Or a couple of glasses of wine before dinner, as I did. These are not responses to nutritional needs; they are responses to established patterns. They aren't necessary to keep us from starving; they just contribute to our daily enjoyment of life. They are habits.

We eat and drink from habit, not from hunger.

Eating from habit means eating without thinking. What you eat isn't usually very important to the habit. You may have an appetite for a wide variety of foods and have preferences that allow you to be flexible in your eating patterns. But when you eat, and how much you eat, can be automatic thoughtless patterns that you follow because of the comfort level they produce.

Habits are formed when your brain learns to respond automatically to a stimulus. A stimulus tells you to eat, and without further analysis, you respond by eating. You get up in the morning and, by force of habit, pour coffee and juice and a bowl of cereal. Or you see that it's 3 PM at the office so you head for the employees' lounge for a soda and a pack of crackers. Or you sit down to dinner and eat much more than you really need, not because you're that hungry, but because dinner usually includes a salad, meat, two vegetables, and a dessert, and you learned as a child to clean your plate. The stimulus of sitting down to dinner leads to the response of eating the full meal – it's a habit.

Forming habits is easy. Each time you respond in the same way to a stimulus, your brain becomes more certain that that response should follow. Before long you don't have to choose a response – it becomes automatic. Having a choice means things could change, and change is uncomfortable. A habit creates predictability, which leads to comfort. It removes the discomfort of having to choose. So you stick to it.

Breaking habits, on the other hand, is extremely difficult. You may know breaking a habit would be in your best interest and want very much to do it, but it's difficult to separate the response from the stimulus. Despite hundreds of "how-to" books, people regularly fail in their attempts to break habits.

The reason they fail is that wanting to do something is an intellectual process, but actually doing is both an emotional and physical process. Deciding that you want to do something is easy because it doesn't, in itself, require change. Actually doing it requires change.

Change is uncomfortable – that's why people hate change. The key to success in changing habits lies in your ability to tolerate the emotional discomfort that is present when you do something new or different. You have to be strong enough emotionally – you need *emotional muscle*.

It requires emotional muscle to do uncomfortable things. The more you change, the more uncomfortable it is, and the more emotional muscle the change requires.

Change can be simple or complex. Going on a commercial extreme-low-calorie diet is complex; you have to plan a whole new eating schedule. Cutting out a couple of smaller items, a couple of hundred calories, is simple by comparison. Whether the change is simple or complex affects the intellectual process of deciding that you want to change; that doesn't require a lot of emotional muscle.

Change can also be easy or difficult. Whether the change is easy or difficult affects the emotional and behavioral processes; the more difficult the change is, the more emotional muscle is required.

Going on one of the commercial diets requires a huge and very difficult change. You no longer can eat as much as you want. You can no longer snack when you normally do. Changing from your normal eating habits to an extremely-low-calorie diet plan disrupts everything you are used to and comfortable with. Most people can manage it for a while, despite the emotional discomfort it causes, because of the promised reward of quick weight loss. It's difficult as well as complex, even if the plan provides meals that are easy and appealing, but you endure it because you know it's temporary. You can see an end to it.

But eating so much less never really becomes a habit. You don't want it to – that would be seriously unhealthy – nor do you expect it to. It's a big discomfort, but it will only last a month or two, so you can stand it.

Eliminating a glass of wine is a much smaller change. It affects only a small part of your daily pattern of eating and drinking. It's both simpler to decide and easier to accomplish. But it still requires leaving a stimulus without a response. It still requires emotional muscle. The "compulsion to completion" that we all share requires doing something, anything, to respond to the stimulus. That makes changing how you respond easier that not responding at all.

James Clear, in his book *Atomic Habits*,[*] expands the stimulus-response process into four parts: a cue, which produces a craving, which brings a response, which yields a reward. The cue starts the process and alerts your brain to

---

[*] *Atomic Habits*, by James Clear. Penguin Random House, 2018.

expect a reward. That produces the second step of the habit loop, a craving, which gives us a reason to act. The craving leads to the response, which satisfies the craving; it also brings us the reward of a craving fulfilled, which in turn reinforces the habit.

Your brain is a reward detector, according to Clear. It continuously scans the environment, evaluating actions that might deliver pleasure or pain, prompting you to seek the former and avoid the latter. When its evaluation proves correct, your brain strengthens the connection between the cue and the reward, setting the habit more firmly in place.

In simplest terms regarding eating habits, the cue may be the sight or odor of something you'd enjoy eating, which creates the craving; you respond by eating it, and your reward is the pleasant experience of eating it and the satisfaction of saying "That was really good, I enjoyed it." Or the cue may be simply knowing that it's time for dinner, so in response, you eat dinner, and the reward is nothing more than that you had dinner as you habitually do.

In order to change your eating habits, you need to break this cycle at some point in the process. There are two ways you can do this. You can eliminate the cue, or you can change the response.

Perhaps the most direct way is to eliminate the cue. If seeing the cookie jar cues your brain to eat a cookie, move the cookie jar out of sight. Hide the cue to avoid the response.

But the cue may not be what you think it is. During the 1890s, the Russian scientist Ivan Pavlov was researching salivation in dogs when they were being fed. He correctly expected that the dogs would salivate when food was placed in front of them. But he soon noticed that the dogs would begin to salivate, not when they saw the food, but as soon as they heard the footsteps of his assistant bringing them the food. The cue, which originally had been the sight of food, had shifted to the sound of the footsteps. Experimenting further, he found that ringing a bell just before the food arrived could produce the same outcome. The dogs' brains had learned that hearing the bell promised that food was forthcoming. So the bell set off the food craving and led to salivation. They responded by eating and were rewarded by satisfying their hunger. Every time they heard the bell, they got to eat; every time they got to eat after hearing the bell, it reinforced the habit pattern. The sight of food, originally the cue, had been replaced by the sound of the bell.

This kind of cue shifting is probably involved in most, if not all, eating habits. You get a cue, not by seeing or smelling something good to eat, but by encountering a stimulus that you have learned will normally precede it. If you have a pre-prandial glass of wine at five o'clock every afternoon, the clock striking five becomes the cue to pour a glassful of wine. If you usually have a bowl of ice cream while you watch the late-night news, the commercial break before the news show becomes the clue, long before you open the freezer.

When I was in the dean's office at Iowa State University, the office manager, Lois, kept a jar of jellybeans on her desk for everybody to enjoy. I needed to go past her desk frequently, and it was easy to help myself. Every time I saw that jar of jellybeans, it was a cue that set off a craving, so in response, I would take a few.

I knew this was a bad habit, and I really wanted to break it. But Lois had been there much longer than I had, and her jelly-bean jar was fully established as an office tradition. I couldn't ask her to remove it.

So I tried to eliminate the cue by making a conscious effort to look the other way when I passed her desk and not see the jellybean jar. That didn't really work, because I still knew that the jellybeans were there, and that became the cue. So the craving began anyway, and as often as not my efforts to ignore the jar failed.

Then I became aware that after I ate the first jellybean, the craving arose even without going near the jar. The jellybeans were "more-ish" – the taste lingered in my mouth, and that was all it took to make my subconscious search for a reason to go back for another one.[*] In a sense, the reward had become the cue.

There was no way to remove that cue except to resist the first jellybean. So I had to find the emotional muscle to eliminate my response to the jelly-bean jar. I had to force myself to pass by it and not automatically – habitually – take a handful.

It wasn't easy, but eventually I broke the habit. I won't try to tell you that I never ate another of Lois's jellybeans; what I did was make them an occasional treat instead of an automatic response.

---

[*] I later learned that my body was probably over-reacting to the sugar rush and producing an excess of insulin, which in turn produced a sugar craving, setting up a recurring cycle. This kind of physiological response may be involved in many addictive habits.

Breaking a habit doesn't mean you never again do something; it just means severing the bond between cue and response. You can have some wine with dinner every night while you're on a cruise, as I have done, or eat twice as much as usual at Christmas dinner as mentioned in Chapter 3. It doesn't become a habit because it isn't a response to a cue that repeats itself in your life. Repetition is an essential part of forming and reinforcing a habit.

Habits are simply processes that you have taught your brain through repetition. If you repeat the same procedure frequently enough, your brain tries to make it automatic once it starts. You have to interfere with that process, either by removing the cue or by changing the response. Removing the cue can be difficult or impossible, as it was with Lois' jellybean jar. Most of the time, it's easier to convert an unhealthy habit to a healthier one by changing the response.

To change the response requires teaching your brain a new response to follow from the beginning cue. Doing that requires concentration and willpower at first, but research shows that it gets easier as it goes along. According to Clear, it generally takes about two months to establish a new pattern, depending on the amount of change required. The good news is that the level of discomfort is greatest at the start of the change. As you continue changing, the discomfort usually lessens significantly. The smaller the change, the easier it will be to establish the new habit.

If I had tried to simply stop having wine with my wife at five o'clock, it would have ruined our enjoyment of a pleasant hour; but we continued relaxing together at the end of the day, just as we always had. The arrival of the end of the workday was the cue, and I didn't want to stop responding to it entirely; I just changed the response to one that didn't include the calories.

You can do that too. Choose something in your daily eating and drinking habit that contains the number of calories you want to lose. Then either eliminate the cue that leads to it or replace the response with something that eliminates that many calories. If it isn't possible to eliminate the cues that tell you it's time for breakfast or lunch or a pre-prandial libation, change your responses to those cues. Instead of eliminating the 550-calorie superburger, replace it with a 300-calorie regular cheeseburger and you'll lose about 15 pounds. Rather than eliminating the 354-calorie serving of French fries, replace it with a 152-calorie bag of chips and lose 13 pounds. Changing, rather than eliminating, requires far less emotional muscle. After a couple of months, you will have established a new response to the stimulus and your new habit will run smoothly.

How do you develop the emotional muscle required to change a habit? Like other muscle, emotional muscle can be built a step at a time. If the change you need is bigger than you can handle, make a smaller one. Instead of initially trying to run five miles, I started by running a mile. I could do that, and once I was used to it, I could increase my distance to two miles, and then bit by bit to five. If you need to, make a smaller calorie reduction that you are comfortable with, and once you've developed the emotional muscle for that change, move to the next level.

A small change will make a big difference. But it must become your new habit. You'll have to have the emotional muscle to stick with it. In the long term, however you choose to do it, you can lose weight permanently only if you reduce your long-term average calorie intake. Not by a lot, but by about fifteen calories for each pound you want to lose.

That's the secret to weighing less long-term. Decide how much you *want* to weigh. Then identify enough changes in your daily diet to let you lose exponentially to that weight. Have the emotional muscle to change your eating habits, either by removing the cue or changing the response.
That works. It did for me. It can work for you.

Appendix A
The Mifflin-St Jeor Equation

The Mifflin-St Jeor group found that the daily Resting Energy Expenditure (REE) is well described by the equation

$$REE = 4.53w + 15.9h - 4.92A + X$$

where w = weight in pounds and h = height in inches.

In order to determine an average individual's total energy expenditure, the Mifflin-St Jeor research team recommended multiplying the REE by an activity factor to account for all energy usage other than basic metabolic functions.

The activity factor can be determined by comparing actual data for calorie consumption with this formula's prediction for the average REE using the average American's weight. The ratio of the two, shown in the graph, is the predicted activity factor. Following primarily the trend of increasing calorie consumption, the activity factor peaks in 2005 and has decreased since; the estimated value in 2020 is 2.246. It seems highly unlikely that the activity level of the average American behaved in this way.

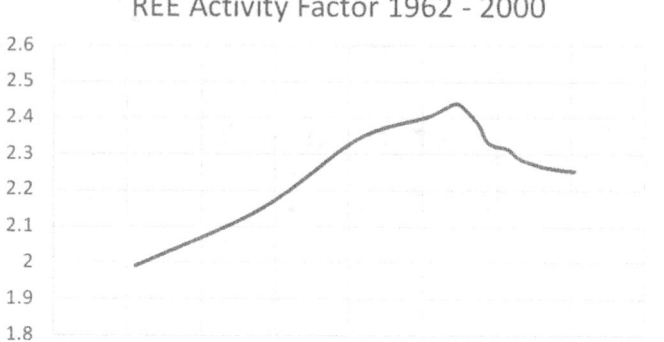

Figure 14. The activity factor required to reconcile REE with TEE, as it varied over time

A better approach would recognize the fact that the calories used in most exercise activities are proportional to weight, but not to the other three factors. That is probably true for all activities as well, so that AEE = λw. Also, it seems reasonable to assume that the TEF is simply proportional to the number of calories digested. If calorie intake and usage are approximately equal, then the TEF is simply proportional to the TEE; I'll assume that it accounts for 10% of the TEE. With those assumptions, the total energy expenditure is given by

TEE = REE + TEF + AEE
= (4.53w + 15.9h − 4.92A + X) + 0.1 TEE + λw

which simplifies to

TEE = $((4.53 + \lambda)w + 15.9h - 4.92A + Y)/0.9$
with Y = 5.56 for men and Y = −179 for women.

The data show that the average American took in about 3434 calories and gained about 0.41 pounds during the time their measurements were carried out. That means about 6 calories were consumed in addition to those required by the TEE, so the value of TEE for an average American at the time of the research can be calculated to be about 3428 calories. If I use that value, along with the average values of weight and height at that time and an age of 45 years, then I can solve for λ and obtain a better result. The result is that the TEE for average Americans in 1990 was given by

TEE = $15.3w + 17.6h - 5.47A + Y$

With Y = +5.56 for men and -179 for women, or equivalently for the average individual,

TEE = $15.3w$ + (700 for women, 981 for men).

Doing the same calculation for 2021, assuming the proportionalities remain valid but using 2021 figures for TEE, weight, and height results in a slight modification to

TEE = $15.3w$ + (714 for women, 977 for men).

Appendix B
The Calculus of Weight Loss

The TEE formula developed in Appendix A can now be used to calculate the time dependence of an individual's weight. I'll do it using the parameters for a woman; for a man, the only difference is a constant additive amount.

Consider a woman whose Total Energy Requirement is a daily number of calories given by the TEE calculated in Appendix A, and assume that she consumes a smaller number of calories C_o than this formula requires. If a pound of fat contains 3500 calories, she will lose weight at a rate $\Delta w/\Delta t$ per day given by

$$\Delta w/\Delta t = -(TEE-C_o)/3500$$

$$= -(15.3w+17.7h-5.47A-179-C_o)/3500 \quad (1)$$

Converting this difference equation to a differential equation yields

$$dw/dt = -(15.3w+17.6h-5.47A(t)-179-C_o)/3500. \quad (2)$$

The terms referring to height (h) and gender (x) are constant. The term A(t), referring to age in years, changes as you age; it is properly described by $A(t) = A_o + t/365.25$, where A_o is the subject's age in years at the beginning of the diet and $t/365.25$ is its daily change. The latter term contributes additional t-dependence to the equation; however, the effect of this second term, compared to the time scales we are considering, turns out to be negligible. If we ignore it, Equation (3) becomes

$$dw/dt = -(15.3w+17.6h-5.47A_o-179-C_o)/3500$$
$$= -(w - w_o)/\tau \qquad (3)$$

where $\tau = 3500/15.3 = 228.8$ days and $w_o = -(17.6h-5.47A_o - 179-C_o))/15.3$.

The solution to this differential equation is

$$w(t) = w_o + (w_i - w_o) e^{-t/\tau}$$

where w_i is the individual's weight at time $t = 0$. This result implies that her weight decreases exponentially from its initial value w_i to an asymptotic value w_o with a time constant $\tau = 228.7$ days and a half-life $T\frac{1}{2} = \tau \ln(2) = 158.4$ days.

With the additional t-dependence of the age term included, the equation is

$$dw/dt = -(w - w_o - at)/\tau$$

where a = (5.47/365.25)/15.3 = 0.000978, and the solution is

$$w = (w_o + at - a\tau) + (w_i - (w_o - a\tau))e^{-t/\tau}$$

It differs from the simpler solution by less than 0.1 pounds over a half-life.

Appendix C
Diet Versus Exercise

Instead of dieting, you can lose weight by exercise, as I did when I started running. In that case, weight loss results from creasing the energy you use, rather than reducing the calories you take in. This is the approach I took when I first started studying this problem after I lost weight thanks to running several miles per day.

Exercise physiologists have measured how much energy different forms of exercise use. The amount is proportional to your weight, which means that exercise also leads to exponential weight loss. For running, the number of calories you use to run a mile is about 0.8 times your weight in pounds. How fast you run doesn't matter much – only how far; it takes about as many calories to run a 5-minute mile as a 10-minute mile.

If you run M miles daily, which adds about 0.80M calories per pound to the calories burned, the differential equation becomes

$$dw/dt = -((15.3+0.80M)w+17.6h-5.47A_o-179-C_o)/3500$$

The only effect is to change the asymptotic weight and the time constant by a factor $(15.3 + 0.8M)/15.3$. If you run a mile per day, you need to include that extra energy use as an additional $0.8w$ in the TEE formulas, so they become

$$TEE = 15.3w + 714 + 0.8w$$
$$= 16.1w + 714 \quad \text{for women}$$
$$TEE = 15.3w + 977 + 0.8w$$
$$= 16.1w + 977 \quad \text{for men}$$

In other words, adding a mile a day changes the proportionality of calories to weight from 15.3 to 16.1 – you require 0.8 more calories per pound per day, which is 5.2% more than you did without running.

If you continue to take in the same number of calories as before you started running, you will lose about 5.2% of your weight for every mile you add to your daily routine. As with dieting, the loss is exponential, but the half-life is shorter by about the same percentage. Running more than a mile a day leads to proportional changes.

The same is true for other forms of exercise. For example, swimming laps for ten minutes about the same number of calories as running a mile. But walking a mile uses only about 90% as much, because walking uses a more efficient gait than running.

The table below shows the approximate number of calories per pound of weight required by either a certain distance or a certain duration of various common exercises, along with the percentage of your body weight you will lose for each.

Activity	Measure	Cals/pound	Weight loss %
Bicycling	5 miles	0.8	5.10%
Running	1 mile	0.8	5.10%
Walking	1 mile	0.7	4.50%
Aerobics	10 minutes	0.6	3.80%
Calisthenics	10 minutes	0.4	2.60%
Elliptical Trainer	10 minutes	0.7	4.50%
Gymnastics	10 minutes	0.3	1.90%
Judo, karate, etc.	10 minutes	0.8	5.10%
Rope Jumping	10 minutes	0.8	5.10%
Stationary Bicycle	10 minutes	0.6	3.80%
Stationary Rowing	10 minutes	0.6	3.80%
Skateboarding	10 minutes	0.4	2.60%
Stair Step Machine	10 minutes	0.5	3.20%
Stretching, Yoga	10 minutes	0.3	1.90%
Swimming laps	10 minutes	0.8	5.10%
Tai Chi	10 minutes	0.3	1.90%
Water aerobics	10 minutes	0.3	1.90%
Weightlifting	10 minutes	0.5	3.20%

Unfortunately, this weight loss lasts only as long as you continue exercising. If you don't, the weight will come back, just as it does when you finish a diet, just as it did to me when I had to stop running

www.ingramcontent.com/pod-product-compliance
Lightning Source LLC
Chambersburg PA
CBHW070649220526
45466CB00001B/364